CW00956280

WOMEN'S
STRENGTH
TRAINING
GUIDE

BARBELL, KETTLEBELL & DUMBBELL TRAINING FOR WOMEN

Get Stronger
Build Lean Muscle
Burn Fat

ROBERT KING

Women's Strength Training Guide
Copyright © 2021 by Robert King

All rights reserved. No part of this publication may be reproduced, distributed,
or transmitted in any form or by any means, including photocopying, recording,
or other electronic or mechanical methods, without the prior written permission
of the author, except in the case of brief quotations embodied in critical reviews
and certain other non-commercial uses permitted by copyright law.

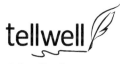

Tellwell Talent
www.tellwell.ca

ISBN
978-0-2288-4976-6 (Hardcover)
978-0-2288-4975-9 (Paperback)
978-0-2288-4977-3 (Ebook)

Dedicated to my mom, Catherine.
Thank you for all your strength.

A Personal Story About my Mother

My mother battled with cancer her whole life. For as long as I can remember, my mother was sick, weak, and taking medications.

Her doctor(s) never once recommend that she eat healthy, exercise, or lift weights.

I tried once to get her to take a multivitamin (she had a handbag full of medications) and she said something like, "Robert, if my doctor thought it was good for me he would tell me to take it."

Seeing this growing up had a big impact on my life to focus on strength, healthy eating, nutrition, and strength training.

My mom had a lifetime battle with cancer. She lost her kidney and her lung; she had numerous heart problems and more. She was a fighter, and after a long battle she came through chemo and made it back home.

Her strength impacted me in countless ways.

Tragically, six months after she beat cancer and chemotherapy, my mom slipped and broke her hip. After that, she never recovered.

What if she had lifted weights?
What if her body was strong enough to take the impact?
What if her bones and muscles were stronger?

I think about these "what-ifs" often...

There are no drawbacks to being stronger. You will never in life feel that being strong was a hinderance. There will be many times in life where we pray for more strength (be it physical, mental, or both).

Being strong is beyond good, especially for women. Being strong is empowering, being strong changes your life, being strong can save your life.

This book is dedicated to my mom, the strongest woman I ever knew.

Thank you for teaching me the importance of strength.

- Coach Robert King

About the Author

I am an entrepreneur, writer, and coach. My current project has been focused on creating and developing an online community for women called Women Who Lift Weights.

For the past 9 years I owned and operated Heavy Weights Training Center, a gym focused on strength training, powerlifting, and body transformation. Most of my clients consisted of women.

Coaching

I have a remarkably diverse background with regards to coaching. I was the Team Canada Head Coach for the 2019 Masters Equipped World Championship that took place in South Africa, the 2019 IPF World Open Championships in UAE Dubai, and the 2019 North American Powerlifting Federation Championships in Costa Rica. I was also assistant coach for Team Canada at the 2019 World Bench Press Championships that took place in Tokyo, Japan.

I have coached thousands of people from varying sports and fitness levels. My major focus has been women's fitness and bikini; recently, I have put more of my attention on powerlifting and strength training.

Writing

I have had the pleasure of writing for some of the top fitness websites and magazines in the world. Some of the magazines include *Strong Fitness Magazine, Men's Health, Women's Health, Inside Fitness, Muscle Insider, The PTDC,* and *Elite FTS*. BigBenchas.com, T-Nation.com, and Schwarzenegger.com are just a few of the websites.

Competing

I have a diverse background in strength sports, martial arts, bodybuilding, weightlifting, and powerlifting. Currently, my focus has been competitive powerlifting. I have competed in more than 50 powerlifting competitions and was selected to represent Team Canada 13 times.

My best accomplishments on the Platform are:

- five-time World Medallist
- three-time Commonwealth Champion
- five-time NAPF (North American Powerlifting Champion)
- Pan Am Champion
- Commonwealth Deadlift Record Holder and National Record Holder
- Multiple Time Canadian National Champion

In June of 2018 I had a total hip replacement. A year and a half later, in October 2019, I competed at the IPF Equipped Masters Worlds Championship in South Africa where I was also the Head Coach for Team Canada. I took home three World's medals that included a bronze in squat, bronze in deadlift, and bronze for overall. It was a lifetime achievement to get on the World's Overall Podium.

Certifications

My certifications include:

- ➤ StrongFirst SFG and SFL
- ➤ Training for Warriors TWF Levels 1 and 2
- ➤ Poliquin Bio Signature 1 and 2
- ➤ CPPS
- ➤ Certified Weightlifting Coach
- ➤ Voted 2014 Personal Trainer of the Year in Orange County, California
- ➤ Black Belt in WTF Tae Kwon Do

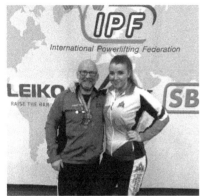

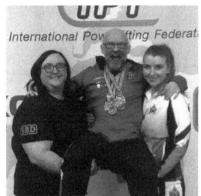

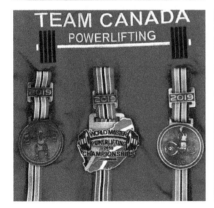

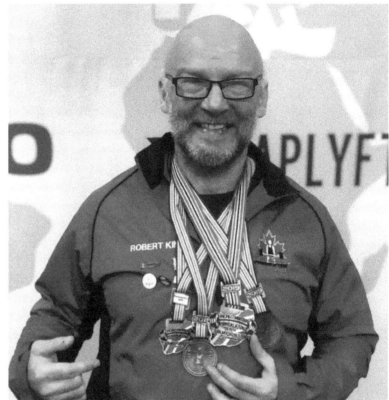

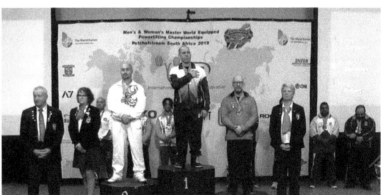

Coach Rob Africa

Acknowledgments

There are many people that have had a huge impact on my life in strength training and coaching, and I'd like to acknowledge a few.

Thank you, Martin Rooney, for our friendship and for showing me a whole other level of coaching and how to truly impact people. You are a life changer.

Thank you, Dan John, for your friendship and for your kind words, guidance, knowledge, and so much more. The SFG weekend in Utah was a life-changing weekend for me and I will always be grateful.

Thank you, Dr. Stu McGill, for your friendship, as well for saving me twice (back injury and hip replacement). Your friendship and knowledge have literally changed my life.

To my Heavy Weights Family over the many years and gyms we had, and to my Elite Training Team: thank you for everything. Being able to lift, train, and have fun with you all has been incredible.

To my many training partners over the years, thank you for sharing The Iron and getting stronger with me. One of my favourite quotations is "Iron Sharpens Iron," and my training partners over the years have helped to sharpen this Iron.

To all the women I have had the privilege and opportunity to coach over the years: thank you. Every single person I have coached has had an impact on me. I am very grateful for that.

Thank you Danielle for your years of work and supporting of Heavy Weights. HW changed many lives, none of it would be possible without you.

Thank you, Nancy and Kevin, from "On The Rock Photograpy", for your help with the pictures. They turned out amazing, I really appreciate it.

Thank you, Rebecca Adams, for everything: our training and your help at World's in South Africa and more. That was the most intense competition experience of my life. Thank you for being there as my training partner, and being in my corner as my Coach and handler. We had a great day/week. I couldn't have done it without you.

To my father for teaching me hard work, dedication to your craft, and to always put in the work. He never missed a hockey game or practice, and I will always be grateful for this support and belief in me.

Introduction

Before we begin, I want to say thank you.

Thank you for reading this book, taking the time to learn how to get stronger and lift heavier, and investing in yourself.

Thank you for trusting in me and thank you for your support.

I am very grateful to have found strength training and lifting weights early in my life. The first time I lifted weights I was about 14 and it completely changed my life forever. Lifting can change you. It empowers you, it rewards hard work, it gives you control. Lifting has changed my life. Along with changing my life it has saved my life in many ways as well.

Lifting weights has helped me though many hard times. When life is good, I trained. When life was not as good, I trained more and I trained even harder.

The Iron has been my teacher, my companion, my friend, and oftentimes my sanity. The Iron always gave me something to focus on, something to improve, something that I could control. The Iron has impacted my mind, body, and soul.

The stronger I got, the harder I trained, the better I felt. After a while, lifting just became part of my day and part of my life. Strength training and lifting weights has impacted my life in so many ways that are hard to describe. Lifting has empowered me to become a better, stronger, happier version of myself.

However, I have always loved the beauty and simplicity of this quotation:

> **"*Strength Serves A Greater Purpose.*"**
> – StrongFirst

Strength goes so much deeper than just how much we lift or how much muscle we have. Lifting weights can change your body, it can impact your mind, and it can leave an impression on your soul.

Thank you for allowing me to share my knowledge and passion with you.

There is nothing that makes me happier than helping others get stronger in the weight room and in life. I hope this book empowers you in many ways, giving you strength, knowledge, and purpose.

Stay Strong.

Coach Robert King

CONTENTS

CHAPTER 1

HOW AND WHY I FOCUSED ON TRAINING WOMEN

I love coaching.

I have been a coach for most of my life now.

I started as a personal trainer back in the 1990s. I did a weekend PT certification course at the YMCA (which was literally across the street from my house).

However, I had been coaching and helping members long before that. In the gym I was "the go-to guy" for all things lifting and strength. This was way before the internet, Google, Amazon, YouTube, etc.

The only resources you had were a few fitness magazines, good books that you could order from bookstores (I worked at one), and many conversations with people in the gym.

Nothing replicates that "floor time" in the gym.

I loved lifting and I loved the gym. It was my passion, my hobby, and my love.

Many years later, around 2013, I took the plunge and decided to expand and open up a gym called Heavy Weights Training Center. At the time I also had a Heavy Weights Supplement Store.

At Heavy Weights Training Center, aka HWTC, we took training and results to a whole different level. What we did for body transformations, strength, and health had "raised the bar" in my province of Newfoundland in Canada.

HWTC was unique and original. There was nothing around like its kind.

Heavy Weights brought the best of everything I knew about strength training, athletic training, healthy eating, fat loss, goal setting, mindset, and much, much more.

HWTC was something unique and different.

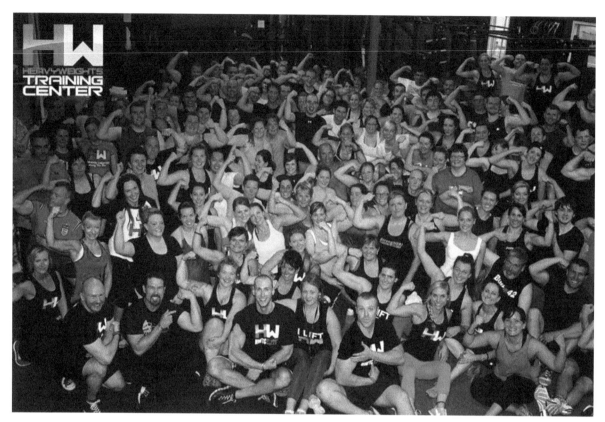

Martin Rooney Fundraiser

We had people say that HWTC was like a cult...they were right: it was a cult...a culture of people looking to lose fat, build muscle, get stronger, feel better, and improve the quality of their lives and surround themselves with like-minded individuals.

We had a very wide variety of members there with female powerlifting athletes ranging from 16 to 72 years of age. We had members training for Powerlifting Nationals and Worlds, and in the same gym we had people taking our fat loss programs like Ripped in 42 and 21 Day Kick Start.

We were like the bar from that show *Cheers*, but instead of a bar we were a gym where everyone knew our name. No matter our goal, we were all there to support and help each other.

Fat loss and body transformations were what got people in the door, but this wasn't my true passion. My true passion was lifting and empowering others to lift.

Along with owning and running the gym I started to get away from coaching our fat loss and transformation programs as we started to develop more lifting-focused programs.

This made me very happy. Weights and lifting were my passion.

We had the best in body transformation results, strength-training results, athletic-training results, and more, all under one amazing roof.

As well, I would always introduce strength training and the benefits of strength training in every single fat loss class.

My goal was to get them in for fat loss but educate them on lifting weights and hopefully get some Iron in their hands.

However, while doing many things at the gym, I started to want to focus more on what I enjoyed most.

The answer was simple: coaching women to get stronger and lift heavier weights. I wanted to help them transform their bodies (and minds) through lifting weights and strength training, not just by cardio and being hungry.

Not only did I love coaching women, but they also loved what was being taught.

A good coach and some Iron can be life changing.

At my gym we did barbell training, kettlebell training, dumbbell training, and much more.

We did squats, deadlifts, bench presses, overhead presses, kettlebell swings, sprints, box jumps, pull-ups, heavy-weighted carries, and more.

You would see sleds, Olympic rings, tire and sledge hammers, and at some points even pushing and pulling my Jeep in the parking lot.

Our female members would get addicted to how amazing it feels to get strong.

My gym became about 75% females. At one point, I think HWTC had over 75 competitive powerlifters, and 50+ of them were female from novice lifters right up to world-level competitors.

What makes this even cooler is that women would join for fat loss programs, and while they were waiting (I did this intentionally on the schedule), they would watch the CST (cardio strength training) class of fit and strong women that I coached.

They would do all the things I posted above and more, but the big focus was that they were all there pushing to lift weights, grow stronger, become more athletic, and have FUN doing it.

Some of these women were not just jacked and strong; some went on to become pro bikini and pro fitness, as well as setting many national powerlifting records and competing for Team Canada, winning world medals, and more.

After coaching these women for a few years, I decided to put most of my coaching energy into coaching women.

Then one day everything in my life changed.

I remember coming home from the gym with this urge, this desire, to create something.

I didn't know what, but I wanted to do something online. The gym can't be my only focus.

I sat down on my couch and did pretty much the exact same thing I had done before.

I asked myself what do I enjoy doing most at the gym all day?

The answer again was simple: coaching women to lift weights and to get stronger, and to transform and empower women through strength training and lifting weights.

Well, if that's what I love, what not take EXACTLY THAT and go online with it to reach even more women, far beyond the doors of my gym in Newfoundland ever could.

What do I enjoy doing?

Coaching women who lift weights.

The name was perfect: "Women Who Lift Weights"

And as they say, the rest is history.

Women Who Lift Weights is now my full-time business, allowing me to coach and reach hundreds of thousands of women every day.

Our Facebook group is incredible, and I couldn't be prouder of how WWLW started, what it has become, and where it is going.

Thank you kindly to all my WWLW members and readers for your support. I am beyond grateful and love what I do.

I love helping Women Get Strong(er) and I am very grateful for what I do.

Yours in Strength,

- Coach Robert King

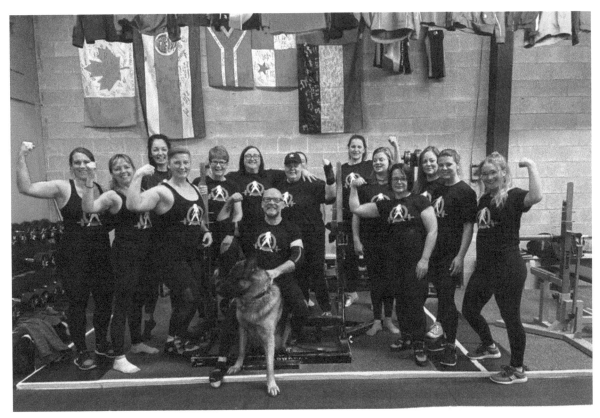

WWLW Team

CHAPTER 2

EIGHT REASONS WHY WOMEN SHOULD LIFT WEIGHTS

Before we start going into the specifics of what you need to know about strength training and lifting weights, we first have to answer the question of why weight train in the first place.

What are some of the benefits for women who lift weights?

There are literally countless benefits of strength training and lifting weights, but I am going to cover what I consider to be the top eight reasons why women should lift.

1. Increased Lean Muscle Mass

The very first reason that tops the list of why you should be weight training is because it will help to increase the amount of lean muscle mass on your frame, which then provides numerous benefits.

First, you have a greater storage house for incoming carbohydrates.
Now, you may be wondering what this means.

Here's what you need to know.

In your body, you have two different storage places for nutrients. You have your lean muscle mass which is where carbohydrates are stored (as muscle glycogen), and then you have your fat cells, which is where dietary fat is stored.

Other nutrients can also be stored in dietary fat as well (such as proteins or carbohydrates) when muscle glycogen is all filled up.

Each time you go to the gym and perform a strength-training workout session, you're going to deplete your muscle glycogen stores. The muscles need those stored carbs for energy; thus, your muscles burns these stored carbs off.

This then means that when you eat carbohydrates later on in your diet, rather than them being shuttled away to the fat cells, they get sent straight to your muscle; thus, you don't gain body fat.

This means you can eat more carbs in your diet and not gain fat. Every woman out there should be rejoicing at this fact right now.

The more muscle mass you have, the more of this storage you also have; therefore, the higher carb your diet can be.

If you're a lover of pasta, brown rice, and whole grains, then you will definitely feel the benefits from strength training.

In addition to having more storage for carbohydrates in the body, when you add lean muscle mass you're also going to increase your metabolic rate.

This means that for every pound of muscle that you build, your body is going to burn off an additional 20 to 30 calories per day.

While it seems like not that much, it adds up. Add 10 pounds of muscle over the course of time, that's an additional 300 calories per day that you can eat.

That's a chicken breast with a cup of rice, that's a bowl of yogurt with some berries and flaxseeds, or, if you're feeling indulgent, that's a small slice of pizza.

This happens all because you built that muscle mass. That additional food will not get converted to body fat as it would if you hadn't built the muscle since you're now burning more calories at rest.

So, as you can imagine, as a method for long-term weight control, building more muscle can't be beat.

Not only can you eat more calories each day without them getting converted to body fat, but you can also eat more carbohydrates and have them stored in a place that is not your fat cells.

It's a win-win scenario for building muscle.

2. Increased Strength Levels

The second reason why you should be working toward a strength-training routine is to enhance muscle strength – as the name suggests. The stronger you are, the less prone to injuries you're going to be and the easier it will be to complete the everyday exercises that you want to be doing.

The important thing to note here is that as you get older, you will begin to lose your lean muscle mass unless you start using it regularly.

Each year, you could lose one to two pounds of lean muscle, meaning your metabolism now goes down each day. You burn fewer calories; thus, you start to see fat gain.

Muscle is very much a 'use it or lose it' type of tissue, so unless you're subjecting them to the overloading stress that weight training provides, you won't be saving those muscle cells.

When you can complete your everyday tasks better, this is going to dramatically enhance your quality of life and you won't feel nearly as fatigued come the end of the day as you normally do.

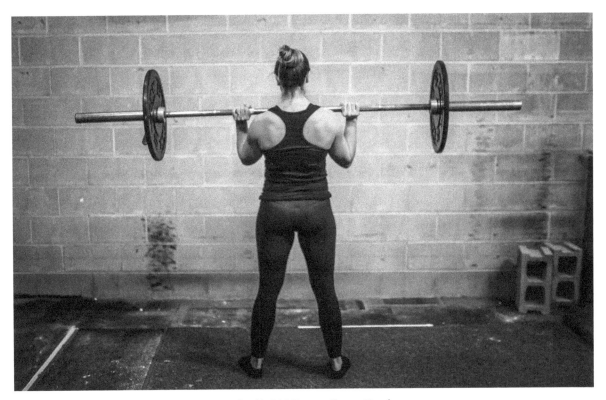

Barbell OH Press Start Back

3. Enhanced Overall Fitness

The third reason to strength train is because of the benefits it will have on your fitness levels. If you're strength training regularly, you'll become more fit. As you get stronger, your resting heart rate will decrease (showing improvements in cardiovascular performance), and you'll be able to sustain a higher intensity exercise over a longer period of time with consecutive weeks of training.

Basically, you'll just be more fit.

If you happen to be involved in a variety of different sporting activities – perhaps you play on a recreational soccer or volleyball team, for instance – you will definitely notice the increase in your fitness level as you go about those practices and games. This increased fitness level is the result of your regular strength-training workout sessions.

Generally speaking, the more fit you are the more you will enjoy those sporting practices as well, so that will be yet another great benefit that you'll notice.

4. Supercharged Fat-burning Ability

The fourth important benefit when performing strength-training workouts is that you'll get a supercharged fat-burning ability from it.

Why's this?

When you strength train, you actually will increase the rate at which the body is able to burn off body fat as a fuel source during rest due to a higher enzymatic reaction in the body.

So basically, rather than burning off glucose as a fuel source when resting, you'll be burning off fat as a fuel source instead.

What's more great news is that not only will your metabolism increase as you perform your strength-training workout sessions, but it will continue to increase for hours after you've completed your workout as well.

If you do a strength-training session in the morning, you'll experience a higher calorie burn all throughout the entire course of the day, making it that much easier to stay lean long-term.

And if your goal happens to be fat loss at this precise moment, then bingo – you've just achieved it with ease.

You'll be quickly burning off loads of calories even while sitting at your desk at work, just because you choose to strength train regularly.

5. Increased Self-Confidence

Another big reason why women should lift weights is this is one form of exercise that will really have a major impact on self-confidence level.

When you're strength training regularly you're going to feel very good about yourself overall as you'll be proud of what your body is accomplishing.

You'll feel empowered by the constant increases in weight you're able to lift and you'll see the positive changes taking place in your muscle shape, tone, and definition.

Each time you walk out of the gym after a hard strength-training workout session, you'll feel as though you're on top of the world.

It sounds a little 'cheesy' but almost all women will find they feel this way. There's nothing like a good strength-training workout to really turn a bad day into a great day. You'll come out of the gym tired yet full of inner energy and feeling great that you're doing something positive for your body.

6. Stress Relief

The next big benefit that you'll get from an intense strength-training session is a high degree of stress relief. You can certainly see stress relief from other activities as well, as there will be certain hormones released from the body after long endurance cardio workouts or you may find you're more at peace with the mind and body after a good yoga workout. However, strength training offers its own form of stress release by allowing you to vent out your frustrations and feel empowered through the act of lifting that heavier weight.

If you're the type of person who often lets stress build up, causing you to become 'angry' in a sense that you just want to hit something, then you will definitely see very good stress-relieving benefits from a good weightlifting workout session.

You'll enter into the gym with a high amount of pent-up hostility and anger. When you come out, this will all be released and you'll feel in control and calm about whatever was bothering you.

7. Challenging and Fun Workout Sessions

The next big reason to add strength-training workouts to the mix is, simply put, they're interesting.

It doesn't take much to realize that cardio sessions are boring.

If you happen to be doing higher intensity cardio sessions then you're slightly better off, as these do typically prove to be a little more interesting, but if you're doing the same old hour-long workout on the treadmill at the gym, you have to ask yourself how long you really will be able to sustain this.

It won't be long before you're dreading every single workout session and just seeking out an alternative – something that offers more mental stimulation while you do it.

Strength training is that alternative.

More importantly, strength training will help you stay with the workout game to begin with. If you're just doing those steady state boring cardio workouts, then it really won't be that long at all before you're falling off them entirely. If you don't switch over to strength training instead, you'll likely just choose to forgo the gym altogether.

Strength training is going to provide the superior option for faster results that interest your mind as well as stimulate your body maximally.

There are so many different exercises that you can perform with strength training, and then there are variations amongst each individual exercise. If you ask yourself how many different ways there are to run on a treadmill, your answer is clear – there is one way to run on a treadmill.

One way that will quickly get boring.

8. Increased Bone Density

I saved the best for last. Since strength training is a weight-bearing exercise – not only are you bearing your own body weight but you're also be bearing that added resistance – this makes it extremely good for strengthening up your bone tissue, causing your bones to stay nice and strong.

Loss of bone density is another important thing that many women have to worry about as they go through the aging process.

If you aren't doing strength-training workouts regularly and taxing those bone cells, eventually they will be lost.

It won't be long before you'll start noticing back, hip, and knee pain and you may even begin to develop osteoporosis or suffer from stress fractures.

By strength training regularly, as well as consuming a diet that is rich in calcium and vitamin D (two nutrients that are very important for strong bones), you can be sure that you're doing everything possible to offset this problem and stay strong into your later years.

When you start suffering bone pain and bone issues, that's when you will struggle to lead the active life that you desire, and this will most certainly have an impact on your quality of life as well.

So, there you have all the top reasons why you should strength train.

Are these reasons enough for you? They should be. Simply put, no other form of exercise comes close to offering so many superior benefits.

If you aren't strength training, you're really missing out. Strength training can be the main focus on it's own, or it can compliment other actitivies and sports.

Hopefully this is enough to get you kick-started with your motivation to head in the right direction. Hopefully you are over any fears that you may become 'muscular or bulky.' While you will likely see some enhanced muscle tone, this will be muscle tone that adds to your femininity and helps you look fitter and more attractive.

Regardless of what your weight happens to be, it's your body composition that matters. You can have two women, both 5'6", one who stands a muscular 140 pounds and 18% body fat and one who stands a very non-muscular 125 pounds and 35% body fat, and they would look like completely different people.

The muscular woman will be lean and svelte and actually look a lot slimmer than the lower-weight one just because of the differences in body composition.

By performing strength training regularly, you will help to tilt your body composition in the lower direction so that more of your body weight is muscle and bone tissue and less is squishy, fat mass.

If you want that firm, toned appearance, strength training is definitely for you.

So now let's move forward and go over some of the main things that many women do wrong when they go about their strength-training workouts.

By getting these out into the open up front, you can be sure that you aren't making these mistakes.

CHAPTER 3

LIFTING LINGO – 35 WORDS AND TERMS YOU SHOULD KNOW

If you are going to lift weights, it's important to also understand certain words, terms, and phrases that play a role in lifting and understanding lifting.

You could call this "lifting lingo."

If you are somewhat new to lifting, you may recognize many of these already. If you have been training for a while, you may know most of them.

However, no matter your level of knowledge, it's well worth reading these terms and getting an understanding of them.

This understanding will make your training better, and it will also give you more clarity and insight in this book as we get into workouts and programming in the later chapters.

Lifting Lingo – 35 Words/Phrases You Should Know (Alphabetical)

AMRAP – "As Many Reps As Possible." This would be doing a set to failure or close to failure with the goal of completing as many reps as possible in the desired set.

Bodybuilding – A competitive sport that is judged by the look of your physique by taking into account leanness, muscular development, symmetry, aesthetics, posting, and more.

Bodybuilding is also known as a type of training where you train to build bigger muscles and improve your overall physique. The end goal here is not performance or the amount of weight lifted like in powerlifting and weightlifting.

Body Part Split – This is how you split your body parts to train during the week. For example, some people will train chest/biceps on one day, back/triceps on another day, then shoulders/legs on the third lift of the week. Some programs require full body lifts for each training session, and some other programs are based on specific pulling or pushing motions (i.e. vertical, horizontal, etc.) instead of focusing on specific body parts.

Body Part Training – Bodybuilders, who are focused on aesthetics over performance, will view the body as individual parts and will train one or two of those parts in isolation apart from the rest of the body in a body part split program.

With these routines, you may be working out five days a week: Monday: Leg Day; Tuesday: Back Day; Wednesday: Shoulder Day; Thursday: Chest Day; Friday: Triceps and Bicep Day.

Circuit Training – Performing back-to-back-to-back exercises (usually two to four different exercises) without resting between exercises.

You may often see this using kettlebells or dumbbells and in bodyweight training. Not often do you see circuits done with barbell training. Although it is possible, it's rarely done. You can use a Barbell in a circuit or complex, but with lifting heavy it's too hard to change the exercises and loads to train in that manner.

Compound Exercice – A multi-joint exercice. Let's think about squats: they use the hip joint and the knee joint. Compound exercises are considered the best bang for your buck.

Concentric – The "positive" phase of the rep. This is the explosive/contraction portion of a rep. On a squat, think of it as the coming out of the bottom of the squat phase.

Contraction – This means the muscle is engaged and contracted to apply force to pull or push a weight. Muscle cells are grouped into motor units, where if one cell in the unit is engaged, the entire group contracts. This is known as the "all-or-none" principle.

Deload or Deloading – A planned period of training time (usually one to two weeks) during a periodization program where intensity, volume, or frequency is reduced to allow for the dissipation of accumulated fatigue. This is done so that proper recovery can be accomplished to allow the stress-recovery-adaption cycle to occur. It is recommended that all lifters take a deload after a heavy training block.

Eccentric – The "negative" phase of a rep. This is the lowering. For example, on a squat the eccentric is the lowering/downward phase.

Failure – The point in an exercise when your muscles are so fatigued that you can no longer perform another rep with strict form.

Sometimes yo u'll see workouts telling you to "perform a set until failure." This means you just crank out as many reps as you can (with strict form) on that set. Usually it's the last set in a workout that you perform until failure.

Sometimes failure occurs even without you wanting it to. If a workout calls for a set of five, but you can only perform four, you've gone to failure.

Forced Reps – Reps that are performed past failure with the assistance of a spotter.

For example, let's say you have a set of five to perform on the bench press and you experience failure at rep three. If your spotter sees that you're struggling, they may grab the bar and lift up on it just enough so you can complete the next two reps before you rack the bar into the pins or uprights of the rack.

Those last two reps are forced reps.

Frequency – How often you train.

Frequency could refer to how often a movement is trained a week, how often a muscle group is trained a week, or how often a workout is performed a week. For example, some programs call for you to work out just three times a week, while others call for you to work out every day.

Full Body Training – Training the entire body in one session because you view the body as a system rather than a combination of individual parts.

For example, some of the programs presented later in this book are more full body training programs than body part splits.

If a lifter is to perform three workouts a week, they will squat, press (or bench press), and pull (deadlift or military press and let's say chin-ups) every single session. You hit both the upper and lower body every single workout. CrossFit also utilizes full body training.

Intensity – The heaviness of the weight being lifted.

How heavy a weight is in comparison to your one-rep max (the maximum amount of weight that you can lift for a given exercise). The heavier the weight, the more intense the lift. Please note that "Intensity" is NOT mental perception of exertion, i.e. "That was an intense workout."

The number for intensity is based off a working number or a percentage of 1 RM.

Isolation Exercices – A single-joint exercice. This can also include exercises that target muscle groups in isolation.

This type of exercise does not involve a big movement of multiple joints. It is an exercise or movement that isolates a muscle group or an exercise that does not require multi-joint movements.

A squat is a compound lift; a leg extension is an isolation exercise.
A pull-up is a multi-joint lift, while a bicep curl is an isolation exercise.

Linear Progression – Only one variable (usually intensity or weight) is incrementally increased per workout to invoke the stress-recovery-adaptation response.

Usually this is done by adding a little more weight to each lift in each workout. Linear progression is best suited for novice lifters. Starting strength is a linear progression program for novice lifters.

Periodization – When you can no longer improve from workout to workout, you become an intermediate and you must begin planned programming. This is called periodization. Periodization includes a variation in volume, intensity, and/or frequency, and it often involves "loading" and "deloading."

Loading – A planned period of training time (usually one to three weeks) during a periodization program of increased intensity, volume, or frequency, where the body is not allowed to fully recover, and fatigue slowly accumulates within the system. This is done so that the body can be stressed enough to elicit an adaptation response, and thus get stronger.

Overtraining – A term used when the body is fatigued and not recovered to perform optimally.

Overtraining occurs when over-reaching stressors occur with too much frequency or with such intensity that the body cannot recover and adapt to better prepare itself for the same stressor. It causes a break in the stress-recovery-adaptation cycle.

Power – Power is strength displayed quickly. It's the ability to contract a large amount of muscle units in a short amount of time. Examples of power in action: standing vertical jump, power clean, sprinting, punching.

Powerlifting – A lifting-based sport consisting of the three main lifts: squat, bench press, and deadlift.

Reps – Everything you do in the gym is a rep. Many people don't realize that strength is practice. Practice is repetitions. When you lift, you don't "work out"; you "practice." There is a big difference.

Reps = Repetition.

Rest Time – How long you take to rest between sets.

This is the amount of time that you rest between each set. Rest time can range from as short as say 10 seconds to as long as 10+ minutes for powerlifters.

RPE – "Rate of Perceived Exertion."

The RPE scale is used to measure the intensity of your exercise. The RPE scale runs from 0 to 10. The numbers below relate to phrases used to rate how easy or difficult you find an activity. For example, 0 (nothing at all) would be how you feel when sitting in a chair; 10 (very, very heavy) would be how you feel at the end of an exercise stress test or after a very difficult activity.

0 – Nothing at all
0.5 – Just noticeable
1 – Very light
2 – Light
3 – Moderate
4 – Somewhat heavy
5 – Not too bad
6 – Feeling a bit heavy
7 – Not bad but getting there
8 – Heavy
9 – Very near max
10 – max, heavy

Sets – A combination of reps in a row will give you a set. A set can be one rep to many reps.

Sticking Point – The portion of the rep that you get stuck at or find hard during a lift. This could be locking out your bench press, the mid-range of a squat, the deadlift lockout, etc.

Split Training – With split training, instead of doing lifts that train the entire body in a single workout, you'll only focus on one major section or movement.

A very common split for strength/performance athletes is two lower days per week concentrating on squats and deadlifts, and two upper body days per week concentrating on presses (press, bench press, dips) and upper body pulling (pull-ups, chin-ups, curls, etc.)

Spotter – Someone to help you during a set, in case you need help lifting or taking the weight. A spotter will also help guide you through a hard rep, give you a lift-off on bench press, and more. A good spotter makes your lifting better for many reasons.

Strength – Force produced against an external resistance. When you're lifting a barbell, the barbell acts as the external resistance. The more force you can produce, the stronger you are. Strength also makes all other physical attributes better.

Strength and tension go hand in hand.

Super Set – Combining two exercises of the same muscle group back-to-back. For example, a bench press followed by a push up.

Tempo aka "Rep Tempo" – The speed at which you complete your sets. For example, let's say you are doing a squat. You lower the weight for three seconds, pause at the bottom for one second, come up fast and hold at the top for one second. This would be a 3-1-X-1 tempo.

Tension – A big word in the strength and lifting community. The more tension (contracting your muscles), the stronger and safer you will be.

Volume – Total weight lifted during your workout.

Generally, you add up all your sets and reps together.

For example, if you squat 185 pounds for five sets of five, you get 185 x 25 (total reps) = 4,625 pounds of volume.

Some people count ALL weights (including warmups) whereas others only count "working sets." A working set is a true hard set, unlike, for example, warming up with the barbell which is still warming up. A working set does not include warmups.

Weight – The amount of weight/resistance that you are using.

The weight is the amount of resistance that you are lifting, such as a 20 lb dumbbell.

Weightlifting – An Olympic sport consisting of two main lifts: the snatch and the clean and jerk.

1RM – Abbreviation for "one rep max."

The maximum amount of weight that you can lift for a given exercise. The easiest way to determine your 1RM is to put weight on the bar until you can't lift it more than once. If you don't want to do that, you can use different calculators out there that try to predict what your 1RM would be based on the weight you can lift for reps.

CHAPTER 4

THE BEST STRENGTH-TRAINING TOOLS

The world of fitness and training has thousands of options for working out and getting results.

You will see everything from body weight exercises to bands to suspension trainers to ropes to ab wheels – the list goes on and on.

Walk into any gym and you will also see an endless variety of machines for lifting and strength. There is a machine for every movement and every muscle.

As well, let's not forget the countless number of cardio machines such as treadmills, ellipticals, rowers, and more.

While all these tools and machines can be used to improve your fitness and training, when it comes to strength training, you can't go wrong with "The Iron."

The Iron is something that is so simple yet so effective that to this day it by far exceeds any other tool when it comes to training for strength and getting results. The Iron has stood the test of time and is by far the best option for strength training and also results.

However, don't let the simplicity of The Iron fool you.

Out of all the modern-day machines for strength training, none of them come close to the results you can get with The Iron, as long as you know how to use it.

Using The Iron for strength training is a skill. Anyone can walk into a gym, sit in a machine, put the pin in place, and use the machine. While this is a form of resistance training, nothing will beat the results and empowerment you get from The Iron when you learn to lift.

While there are many tools that you can use to develop your strength, your body, and your mind, there are three tools that I consider to be the foundation of strength training: the barbell, the kettlebell, and the dumbbell.

These three training tools are the foundation of strength training and developing mental strength.

Each tool has its own pros and cons, its own area of development and uses.

Knowledge of just one of these tools can improve your strength and results more than any machine or gadget on the market today.

Add in knowing two or three of these, and you have unlimited exercises, combinations, and program options.

The Iron is a never-ending quest of strength, development, and improvement. The more you think you know, the more you realize there is so much more to know.

"I have found the Iron to be my greatest friend.
It never freaks out on me, never runs.
Friends may come and go. But two hundred
pounds is always two hundred pounds."

—Henry Rollins on The Iron

CHAPTER 5

THE BARBELL

A Personal Story About the Barbell

I am not sure when it happened, but there is no denying that it did happen.

I got bitten by The Iron and fell in love with the barbell.

During my first few years of training, my primary focus was to improve my martial arts abilities. I didn't care to get bigger; I just wanted to perform better and be faster. Getting bigger or stronger wasn't the goal.

After that, I started getting into the bodybuilding scene.

We always trained with heavy weights and power lifts (squat, bench, deadlift). I even competed in both powerlifting and bodybuilding in 1999.

Then, in 2000, my life was changed.

I was pulling a heavy sumo and it got stuck at about my knees. It stayed stuck and I kept pulling…I was not going to give up…then BANG. It felt like someone shot me in the back.

I had to get help to walk to my house across the street from the YMCA. My lower back was never the same until 2013.

In 2013, I met Dr. Stu McGill. I started to rehab my back, and I started to get a better understanding of strength training, technique, tension, movement, and more.

I earned my way back to the barbell and then fell in love with The Iron and the barbell again.

There is no other tool that I love in training more than a barbell.

Fast-forward from 2000 when I injured my back, and I made my way back to the platform, back to competing, and beyond.

In 2014, I made Team Canada for the IPF World Championships in South Africa. It was a big learning curve on so many levels. My back was good but was still not 100%.

The following year, in 2015, I competed again with Team Canada at the IPF World Championships in Finland.

I had a GREAT day on the platform going 8/9, and walking away with a bronze medal in Deadlifts and also a Commonwealth Deadlift Record (252.5 kg at 83 kg M1 division).

To say I was happy does not do it justice. It was one of the best experiences and accomplishments of my life.

The Iron and the barbell taught me many lessons: I learned respect; I learned resilience; and I learned that the human body is capable of almost anything with the right training and mindset.

The barbell changed my life in so many ways and it will be a part of my life forever.

Now, as a coach, I love to introduce to barbell training. There is nothing that is more empowering than a heavy barbell on your back or in your hands.

The Anatomy of the Barbell

The barbell is the single most important piece of equipment in any gym. There are many different barbells, but they all share some common parts including sleeve, collars, and knurling. Olympic barbells add spinning sleeves and bearings to this. Most barbells are 6' to 7'2 long and 25 mm to 32 mm thick and can handle plenty of weight for most lifters.

As you can see below, there are quite a few parts to a barbell.

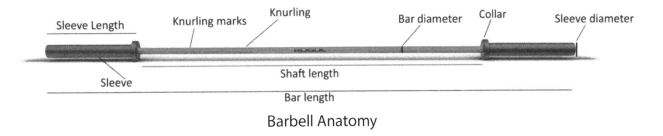

Barbell Anatomy

Parts of the Barbell

Shaft: The rod that makes up most of the length of the barbell.

Sleeves: At both ends of the shaft there are sleeves attached. Weight plates are loaded onto these sleeves.

Bearings: The bearings aren't visible from the outside, but they sit between the shaft and the sleeves. This allows the sleeves to spin independently from the shaft.

Collar: The collar is not a separate part; it is integrated into the sleeves. The collar is a thicker part that prevents the weight plates from sliding onto the shaft.

Knurling: The knurling is the cross-hatch pattern in the shaft. It's not a separate part but it's important. It helps you keep a grip on the bar in all circumstances.

Knurling marks: The knurling usually has rings in it. For home use they're useful for gripping the bar the same way in every exercise. Their real use is for competitions.

Dimensions: Some of the most important features of any barbell are the dimensions. These are not the only features but they're a good place to start. There are three dimensions you should be aware of with barbells.

Barbell Length: Barbells come in many different lengths. All lengths have different purposes and are suitable for different situations.

Barbells range from 4' to 8' in length. The most common size is 7'2 feet but others are commonly seen as well.

The official Olympic men's barbell length is 86.75 which is where the 7'2 standard comes form. Women's official barbells are 79.13" long. Those two are the most common in gyms around the world for general purposes. For home gyms, those lengths are perfectly fine as well, although a 6' long one would also be suitable.

FYI, Olympic barbell can mean that it's built to Olympic standards, but for most cheaper bars it just means that there are 2" spinning sleeves at the ends. More on that later.

It's important that you have enough length on the bar so you can take all the hand positions you want while also being able to load up all the weight plates you need. If you're a smaller person with shorter arms and a narrow frame, you can get away with using a shorter barbell since your reach isn't as wide. If a barbell fits on a power rack, it's going to be wide enough for all exercises.

The vast majority of power racks have their hooks 48" apart. To use the bar on a power rack, you'll need at least 50" of shaft length. That means that some 6' bars fit and others don't depending on how they have been made shorter. For bars that are used outside the rack, you can use whatever works for you.

For general use in a home gym, a bar that's 6' to 7'2 long will work fine as long as it fits on the power rack.

Barbell Diameter: The next important dimension is the diameter of the bar. Like the length, there are quite a few different diameters available. What are the different diameters and what are they used for?

Normal barbells have a shaft diameter that ranges from 25-32 mm. The two most common diameters are 25 mm and 28 mm. In official competitions, the 25 mm bars are used by women while the 28 mm bars are used by men. This is because women have smaller hands in general and the men's bar is often too big to get a good grip. The hook grip is especially difficult on a thicker bar.

30 mm and 32 mm bars are most often used for powerlifting-style squats. The extra thickness makes the bar stiffer and makes it have less whip, and this helps at the bottom of a squat. It's also a really easy way to make a bar stronger.

Barbell Weight: The vast majority of barbells you'll see in gyms weigh 20 kg or 44 lbs. Shorter and thinner bars often have a weight of 15 kg. The lighter and thinner bars are often used by women.

Women's Barbell: Some brands offer different-sized barbells for men and women. For women, the official diameter is 25 mm at a weight of 15 kg. Since women tend to have smaller hands than men, the smaller diameter helps with grip. Thinner bars have less metal and this causes them to be lighter.

In the sport of powerlifting there is no women's barbell. There is only a standard 20 kg barbell with a standard diameter of 30 mm or 32 mm and length of 7'2 feet.

The Benefits of Barbell Training for Women

There are countless benefits of barbell training for women, but I am going to do my best to summarize what I consider to be the most important reasons.

Barbell Training Improves Overall Strength and Full Body Strength

One of the most powerful things about barbell training for women is that it helps them get stronger more than any other training tool.

Lifting weights and strength training will improve overall full body strength, and a barbell is in my opinion the best tool for this.

Unlike most machines that create somewhat isolated strength, the barbell is a great tool to teach not only strength, but full body strength.

There is a big difference between being strong on a machine versus being strong overall.

Unlike using machines in a gym which often target individual muscle groups, the barbell when used correctly turns your whole body into steel. It creates full body strength from head to toe and forges a body of iron. Many women may have a strong leg press or lift heavy with a certain machine, but if you want to be really strong you must learn and master the basic lifts. For this you need the barbell.

While any type of strength training has benefits, the barbell takes strength training one step further than pretty much every other tool.

Barbell Training Can Help Build Lean Muscle

One of the biggest things I have noticed when it comes to coaching women is that when they start strength training with a big focus on the barbell, they completely change their body.

When women start lifting, their physique changes. They start to build lean and powerful muscles. Oftentimes this initial change can happen very fast. Women can literally change their physique in six months with the combination of strength training and proper nutrition.

Body transformation is one thing, and building a few pounds of muscle is one thing.

But don't caught up in the belief that you are going to "bulk up" or "look like a man" after a few weeks or months of lifting weights.

If only it were that easy...

With less than one-twentieth of the testosterone of men, building muscle for a woman is not an easy task.

However, with proper strength training, nutrition, and rest, women are able to build quality lean and strong muscle.

Again, don't be concerned about getting "bulky" or "manly"; that will not happen. I will cover this in more detail in Chapter 13.

Barbell Training Can Enhance Fat Loss and Calorie Burning

Another big benefit of barbell training is that it will impact your metabolism and improve fat loss and calorie expenditure.

After coaching thousands of women, I can honestly say that when a woman is able to lift heavier weights and get stronger, in return they earn the right to eat more calories. This makes them (and their coach) much happier ☺.

But you have to "earn" the right to eat those calories. That's where strength training and lifting weights comes in.

Often women are always thinking in terms of eating less and burning calories.

This is a wrong mindset to have. It's a "losing" mindset. "Eat Fewer Calories" and "Train More" aka "Burn More Calories."

While this is somewhat true, there is a better and happier and healthier approach: get stronger.

When you start to lift and get stronger from barbell training, it becomes important to eat to feed your training and recovery.

This is a switch from the common "Burn More" and "Eat Less" theory.

The barbell is a great tool to improve fat loss and calorie expenditure. In my opinion, it's far superior to most forms of "cardio" and machines.

By focusing on getting stronger, building more lean muscle, and improving athletic performance, your metabolism can change dramatically. This can change your body much faster than lowering your caloric intake and burning more calories.

Barbell Training Can Decrease Osteoporosis

One of the biggest benefits of barbell training for women (especially as they age) is the impact it has on osteoporosis.

The barbell plays a large role in this because of the amount of weight that you are able to lift.

More than any other strength-training tool, the barbell will allow you to lift the heaviest weights and loads which in turn causes more "good stress" on the body. In return, this helps prevent and lower osteoporosis.

While there are many tools that can be used for strength training, the barbell can apply the heaviest loads along with great movements. This is win/win situation for impacting osteoporosis.

Barbell Training Can Decrease Stress

Fitness overall is one of the best things we can do to help with stress. There are thousands of studies and examples proving this to be true.

Lifting weights and strength training play a huge role in stress relief. For some, this reduces stress more than any other exercise.

Speaking for myself, I can say I am never happier (and less stressed) than after a heavy barbell workout. This brings me happiness and reduces my stress immensely.

I can speak from experience after coaching thousands of women that for some, the barbell may bring the greatest source of stress relief.

Barbell Training May Help Reduce Injuries

Another benefit of barbell training is reduction of injuries. Being strong overall will make you more durable and "tempered."

A strong body is a harder body to break and is more resistant to injuries, aging, and life.

Barbell Training May Improved Cardiac Health

While most people associate "cardio" with improved cardiovascular health, the barbell and strength training also play a huge role on improving the cardiac system.

Squatting, deadlifting, putting weights overhead, and other exercises like these will make your heart work.

And if you still have doubts, try a set of 20 rep squats with some heavy weights, or try German Volume Training, and then we can talk ☺.

Barbell Training May Improve Confidence and Sense of Well-Being

One of the most positive and undervalued aspects is the impact on a woman of barbell training and the feeling of getting strong.

Once you start lifting, there is a huge impact on your confidence and overall sense of well-being.

Feeling strong and lifting heavy weights empowers you and improves confidence. I have seen countless women walk into my gym with poor posture, head down, and low confidence.

Months of strength training and barbell training can positively change a woman physically and mentally.

Lifting Weights and Getting Stronger is a Very Empowering Feeling for Women

I always go back to the deadlift for confidence.

To properly complete a deadlift, you have to stand tall with shoulders back, chest up, and head high while holding a heavy-loaded barbell that you picked up from the floor now in your hands.

Physically and psychologically, the deadlift is a very powerful thing.

The same feeling can be applied to putting weight overhead with lifts and exercises like the clean and jerk, the snatch, the push press, and the military press.

"There is something simple and powerful about lifting heavy weights off the floor and putting heavy weights over your head."

—Coach Rob King

The Drawbacks of the Barbell

As much as I love the barbell more than any other tool, I must confess something.

I do feel that the barbell, more than any other tool, has the ability to hurt and cause injury.

This is why it's imperative to learn correct technique and always respect the weights and the barbell.

Barbell Training May Cause a Higher Risk of Injury When Not Using Proper Form

When using a barbell, you are training with a weight/load that may involve using more weight than most other strength-training tools.

While there is always a possibility of getting hurt or injured when using a strength-training machine or another strength-training tool, the loads on the barbell are usually much higher.

The barbell is a double-edged sword. It's an incredible tool when you know how to use it, but if you use too much weight with bad form, you have a higher chance of injury.

It's important to learn proper barbell lifting techniques, proper form, and exercises (when possible from a qualified coach or certification).

Proper Knowledge of Lifting Techniques

The barbell also requires technique, coordination, balance, and timing.

If we look at say a deadlift versus a leg press, it's pretty clear which lift is more demanding on technique and skill.

With a barbell there is a higher level of learning and technical proficiency, along with heavy loads.

Unless you lift with proper technique and form, this can be a bad mix.

When lifting the barbell, perfect form is always a must.

Limitations of the Barbell

One of the biggest limiting factors of the barbell is that it is not very moveable in certain motions.

For example, with the bench press your wrist will always be in a semi-fixed position. This is the same with the squat and the deadlift, etc.

However, when you look at a kettlebell or a dumbbell, you have the ability to move your wrists and other joints and aspects of the body around the tool.

The barbell is a wonderful tool for training and strength, but it's not as forgiving as some other tools.

Another limitation of the barbell is the weight always being equal and on the outside of the body. Rarely would you use uneven loads in training (it can be done but is risky and for advanced lifters).

The barbell is always loaded on the outside, unless you are doing barbell variations like landmine and single arm exercises.

What About Weightlifting?

Weightlifting is a sport that is composed of the snatch and the clean and jerk.

While that simple sentence explains what weightlifting is, it does it no justice to the level of skill and complexity of these lifts.

Author's Note: Please note that I have not included any weightlifting exercises or weightlifting accessory exercises on this list.

While I have the utmost respect for these lifts and think they are great lifts and exercises, the reasons for not adding them are twofold.

1. The complexity of the lift makes it difficult for most people to learn "relatively easily."

2. Most people who do not move well enough will have trouble with these lifts and exercises. If you are not mobile through the hips, shoulders, wrists, and more, then these exercises have a much higher risk/reward ratio.

While I have the utmost respect for these lifts and I have also competed in and coached weightlifting, for the simplicity of the average person looking to learn more about strength training and barbell training I find these exercises are not for most women.

However, if you move well, you can find a great coach, and you have a solid base of squatting and overhead pressing, then weightlifting may be a great option for you.

Being a powerlifting coach and Team Canada powerlifting coach I am clearly biased toward powerlifting.

CHAPTER 6

TOP FIVE BARBELL EXERCISES

Top Five Barbell Exercises

1. The Barbell Back Squat

2. The Barbell Deadlift (Conventional and Sumo)

3. The Barbell Bench Press

4. The Barbell Overhead Press

5. The Barbell Lunge (Forward and Backwards)

#1 The Barbell Back Squat

How to do a Barbell Back Squat: I like to break down the barbell squat into four simple and very important steps.

1. The Setup

Face the bar and be sure the bar is centred and everything is ready to go (I always double-check my bar before I lift).

Have the bar positioned at clavicle height (high bar) or sternum height (low bar). These heights are approximate as every lifter will have their own preference.

Grab the bar tightly with a medium grip. As a simple rule of thumb, try to pull your hands as close to your shoulders as possible. This will help create an area for the bar. Hand grip width will be a very individual factor.

You can use a full grip with thumbs around or go with a thumbless grip.

Do NOT put the bar on the little bony spot on the back of your neck ☺.

Place the bar on your upper back by dipping under the bar. Try to lay the bar on top of the trapezius (high bar) or the shelf of the scapula (low bar).

Try to get very tight with the barbell in the rack; this is very important.

Before the bar comes off the rack, you want maximum tension/stiffness throughout the whole body. The more weight, the more tension.

Consider your setup as being as important as your first rep.

2. The Unrack/Walk Out

Move your feet under the bar. Unrack it by straightening your legs. Be sure to stand the weight up by using your legs and hips, not your lower back.

Make sure you take a big breath into your belly and brace your core hard before you stand up the weight. You will keep core stiffness throughout the unrack and walkout.

Step back slowly with control and set your feet about shoulder-width apart, or a little wider. Every lifter will find their own optimal squat stance over time.

The goal of the unrack and walk out is minimal movment. Try to do it in 2-3 steps.

Once you have walked back, set your feet (I always like to think of my feet gripping and pulling apart the floor). Once your feet are set, be sure to squeeze your quads and glutes and lock your knees.

Have your toes pointed straight ahead or slightly pointed out (this will be very individual as well).

You are now ready to start the squat.

3. The Squat

Take a big breath and brace your core in a 360-degree fashion. Keep stiffness in the whole trunk (not just the front abs).

Initiate the squat with a very small hip hinge and let your upper body move slightly forward.

Some people like to think break the hips first, then the knees. Others like to go with hips and knees breaking the same time.

Either is fine; practice both and find what works and feels best for you.

As you start to "sit back" be sure to push the knees out as well.

Be sure to keep the knees over the toes while thinking also about "spreading the floor."

While maintaining upper body stiffness, squat as deep as you can to a level that is comfortable for you.

How deep you squat will depend on numerous factors such as mobility, injuries, footwear, age, hip anatomy, competition federations, and much more.

A simple goal is to try to achieve parallel or a little bit lower than parallel, or full depth depending on factors and the goal(s) of the squat.

Finish your rep first by holding the bar with locked hips and knees at the top.

Repeat each rep with a goal of lifting perfection and repetition.

The goal is not to get tired.

The goal is to get stronger and better.

4. The Walk In / Re-rack

Then walk forward and re-rack is a very neglected yet important part of the squat.

Oftentimes many squats go wrong and people get injured not during the squat, but during the re-rack.

Be sure to walk in by yourself or when possible have a spotter(s) help you re-rack the barbell.

Lower the barbell into the racks using your legs and hips. Do not lean forward or bend through the lower back.

Before you release tension/stiffness, be sure that both sides of the barbell are racked securely and safely.

The set is not over until the barbell is racked back safely in the rack.

Safety Note: When possible, try to squat in the power rack for maximum safety. Set the horizontal safety pins so they can catch the bar if you fail to squat it. Don't squat in the Smith machine with the bar attached on rails. Machines are ineffective for gaining strength and muscle. If it's all you have, then by all means use it, but when possible use a standard barbell and a squat rack or power rack.

If you do not have access to a power rack, try to have a good spotter(s).

If you do not have access to a power rack or spotters, it is very important you learn how to "ditch" or "bail" a squat safely. This can be done with practice just like doing a barbell squat.

Safety is paramount when squatting with a barbell.

Coach Rob's Tip:

The barbell back squat is the king of strength training and barbell exercises. Be sure to focus on technique as it sets the stage for the rest of the barbell lifts.

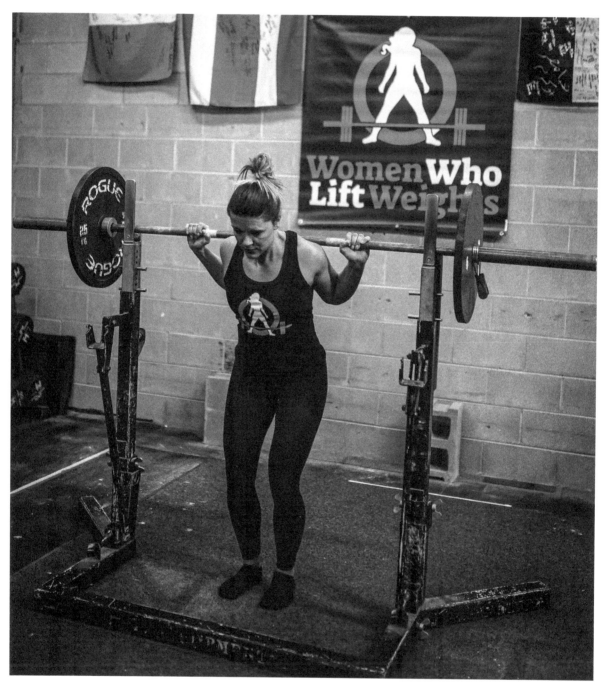

Squat Start Rack

High Bar versus Low Bar

It's important to note there are two kinds of barbell back squats: the high bar squat and the low bar squat.

Bar Position

With a high bar squat, the barbell is placed on the trapezius muscle (aka the traps).

With a low bar squat, the barbell is placed lower on the centre of mass of the mid-back. Usually, the bar in this situation will set on the "shelf of the scapula."

Squat Type

High bar squats are usually known as a knee-dominant squat. The focus of the squat, due to the bar position and weight distribution, is more toward the lower half of the quads, thereby making this a "quad-dominant" squat.

As well, the high bar will really target your core/midsection.

I call the front squat a quads-and-core-focused squat.

Low bar squats are more of a full-body movement with a bigger emphasis on the muscles of the hip and upper back. Because the bar is lower on the back, in the bottom of the squat the weight is centred back more and closer to the centre of gravity.

Usually with low bar you can lift more weight, but it is also generally a bit harder on the shoulders, elbows, and wrists.

Both high bar and low bar squats offer benefits and are good exercises depending on your training goals.

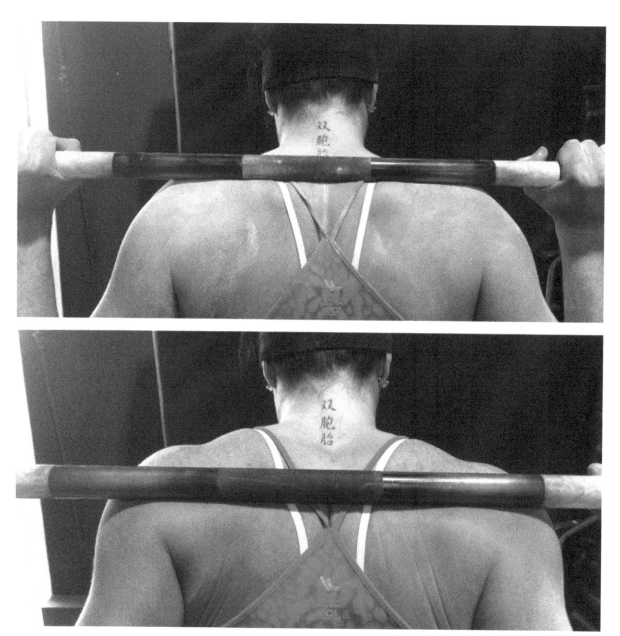

High Bar vs. Low Bar

#2 The Conventional Deadlift

How to do a Conventional Deadlift

The conventional deadlift is one of the simplest yet most complex barbell exercises.

I mean it's just a barbell on the floor with weights you pick up, right?

Well not really...actually not even close.

Conventional deadlifts are in many ways the backbone of powerlifting, strength training, and lifting weights.

Learning proper technique in a conventional deadlift is not only necessary for strength, performance, and building muscle, but also for reducing chance of injury.

Out of all the barbell exercises, it's the conventional deadlift that usually causes the most injuries.

On the flip side, the conventional deadlift is one of the best exercises to build full body strength and injury resilience.

When it comes to back injuries with conventional deadlifts, it's important to know it's not the deadlift that causes problems, it's how you deadlift.

A deadlift injury usually comes down to 3 things:

1. Poor Technique
2. Too Much Load
3. Read #1 and #2 again

There are some times that you may hurt your back if you have some type of pre-existing problem, but for the most part the injuries and setback are caused by improper technique and just using too much weight.

A simple fix for this is to always rely on perfect technique, and never lift to the point where form breaks down.

Three Important Things Before We Get to the Deadlift

1. Deadlift barefoot or in shoes with a minimal flat sole. You do not want to deadlift in sneakers or running shoes. As well, avoid an elevated heel when possible.

2. It's important to learn a proper hinge in order to do a conventional deadlift.

3. Always respect the barbell and the weight on the barbell.

The Conventional Deadlift

I like to teach the conventional deadlift in three simple steps.

1. The Setup

Step up to the barbell and assume about a shoulder-width stance. Have your toes pointed straight ahead or very slightly pointed out (this will be a very individual thing).

Once you step up to the barbell, you want your shins to be about one to two inches away from touching the barbell. Again, this is a very individual thing based on many factors.

When starting out, a simple tip is to look down and have the barbell be above your laces if you were wearing sneakers.

When you look down, use landmarks on the bar to make sure that your feet are centred on the bar.

Be sure to set your feet using a tripod foot with a base of support on the ball of the foot, the pinky toe, and the heel.

Once you set your feet, get your balance and now it's time to get your air.

Take a big breath into your stomach and create a brace of your trunk. You should be creating a 360-degree brace going the full way around your midsection.

Take a big breath, and then start to descend to the bar.

As you descend, never ever just bend over and pick up the bar. This is a big mistake a lot of new lifters make.

Instead, be sure to initiate the movement with a proper hip hinge by sitting the hips back with a slight knee bend (soft knees) and letting your upper body come forward.

Push your hips back as far as you can, loading up your hamstrings and the muscles of the hips.

It is very important to maintain a "neutral" spine throughout the hinge.

As you push your hips back, you also need to start bending your knees, allowing them to come forward. This bend of the knees will be very individual for each lifter for numerous reasons such as anatomy and levers.

Generally, a shorter lifter will have more of a forward knee bend, while a taller lifter may require less knee bending.

As you lower to the barbell, think of your body as being a coiled spring, compressing energy.

Lower until you reach the barbell. Once you are able to touch the barbell, grip the barbell as tightly as possible.

Once you grip the barbell, think about squeezing your lats as hard as possible. A simple cue for this is to think about closing off your armpits.

Pull your shoulders back and down (think anti-shrug) and maintain stiffness/tension throughout the whole body.

Keep your arms straight and think of them as being like long hooks. Do not lift with the arms; hold and create tension with the arms.

If at any point someone were to come and push any part of your body, you would be rigid and not easy to move. This is creating full body tension.

Once you have your hands on the barbell and you are creating tension, then be sure to pull yourself into the barbell.

This is known as a "wedge," and it is also known as taking the slack out of the bar.

The bar should rise to the top of the plates to make a "clink," yet the barbell does not move off the floor.

Think of using a jack to lift a barbell: you place a jack under the barbell, you get it in tight, and then you lift the barbell off the floor.

Keep your head with eyes on the horizon or eyes slightly down.

This takes us to step 2.

2. The Deadlift

A proper deadlift starts with a proper setup, and now that we have done everything correctly, we are ready to begin the deadlift.

Once you have created a strong wedge and pulled yourself into the bar, your next step is to focus on pushing the floor away from you. Do not pick up the weight.

Picking up the weight off the floor is one of the most common conventional deadlift errors.

Instead, be sure to stay tight and push the floor away from you. For the most part, the initial "first pull" of the deadlift (floor to knee) is mostly a push using your quads.

Once the bar starts to move off the floor, be sure that your shoulders and hips rise at the same time.

The barbell should be as close to your body as possible and, if possible, maintaining contact with your body as it travels up the shins and then the quads and the hips.

As the bar starts to travel off the floor, you want to create a strong contraction of the glutes/hips pushing them into the bar.

Once the bar crosses the knees, you are pulling the bar hard with your hamstrings and upper back and forcefully contacting your hips into the bar. This is often referred to the "second pull."

Finish the deadlift by standing tall with chest up, shoulders back, hips locked, knees locked (but not hyperextended), and glutes squeezed with your body in a neutral position and standing with full control of the weight.

Eye position can vary from person to person. Some like to finish the lift looking down, some maintain an eyes-on-the-horizon finish, some look straight ahead, and some even look up with eyes to the sky.

There is no real "best" position for this. Find the one that feels best for you. For the most part, I like to teach lifters to let their eyes and head go wherever feels natural for them.

Be sure to "own the lift" at the top of a lockout on conventional deadlifts.

3. The Eccentric (The Lowering)

The lowering of the deadlift is often the part that ends up hurting people the most.

This may be a result of improper lowering mechanics and lack of maintaining proper tension.

It is very important in the lowering process to first move from the hips, and to not bend from the lower back.

If you go to lower the weight and move from the lower back first, then you will end up at some point causing back discomfort, pain, or injury.

It's very important to maintain tension at the top of the deadlift and reverse it down by initiating with a top-down hip hinge.

Be sure to push the hips back into a hip hinge and do not bend from the lower back.

Maintain sufficient full body tension throughout the lowering until the barbell is back on the floor.

Coach Rob's Tip:

Mastering the conventional deadlift requires perfect practice. It's a mixture of creating full body tension, learning a proper hip hinge, and developing perfect lifting technique.

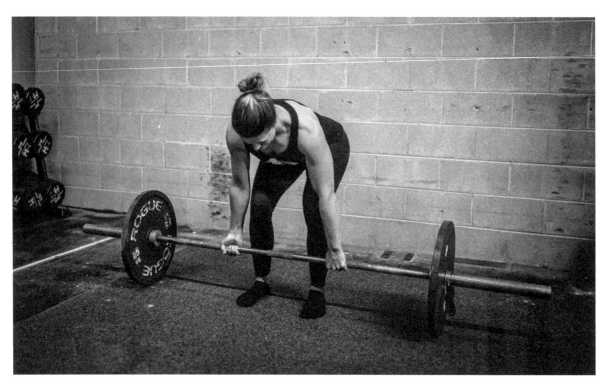

Conventional Deadlift Start

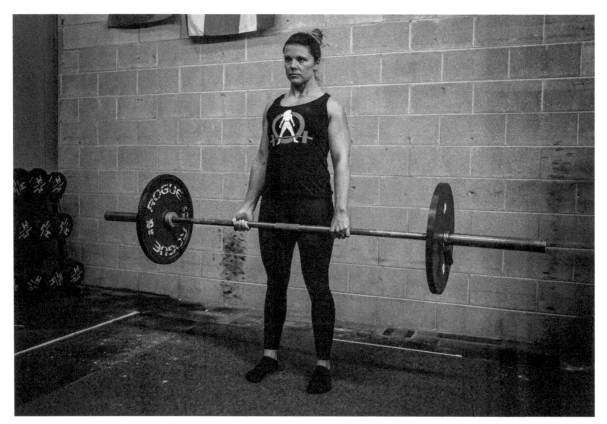

Conventional Deadlift Finish

The Sumo Deadlift

How to do a Sumo Deadlift

I like to break the sumo deadlift down into three components.

Step 1 – The Sumo Deadlift Setup

Step up to the barbell and take a wider-than-shoulder-width stance. Everyone's stance will be different and unique to them, but for the most part have a wider-than-shoulder-width stance with your toes pointed slightly out.

An easy point to remember is to always think about sumo wrestlers with their wider stance and their feet and toes pointed out in a strong and powerful stance.

Look down and make sure that your shins very close to the barbell. It can be anywhere from almost touching the barbell to about one inch away. Have your feet and toes slightly pointed out.

If possible, use a landmark on the bar like the rings to make sure that your feet are even on both sides.

Once your feet are set and you are close to the barbell, start by pushing your hips back and opening your knees out. Think of opening the hips, knees, and groin and try to "sit back" and slowly lower yourself toward the bar.

I like to take a big breath into my belly and brace my core here. More information on breathing and bracing can be found below.

Have your arms go straight down from your shoulders. They should not be too close or too wide; straight down is usually the best option.

Lower yourself toward the barbell. With "long arms," keep sitting your hips back. Open the knees and also be sure to "spread the floor" with your feet. Imagine that you are standing on two pieces of paper and you are trying to push them apart.

As you lower to the barbell, try to maintain a "neutral spine" as much as you can. You want to create and maintain upper body tension and stiffness throughout the whole process.

Once you are able to get your hands on the barbell, you want to grip the bar as hard as possible. A strong grip will improve tension throughout the whole body. Having a strong grip is also very important for holding on to the deadlift. For now, let's focus on having a "double over" grip where both palms are facing toward you.

As you grip the barbell, be sure to think about "breaking the barbell" in your hands. You don't want to just hold the barbell; you want to try to crush it.

Once you grip the bar tightly, try to get your lats and upper back tight. A great way to think about this is to squeeze your armpits. It sounds somewhat funny. Imagine that if someone were to try to tickle you, there is no way you would let them. This will help get your lats tight.

Now that you have set your hips back and pushed your knees out, be sure to keep the hips as high as possible. This is not a squat, it's a high hinge, so keep the hips as high as possible.

The next step is very important and often neglected, and that is creating a "wedge" and pulling yourself into the bar. You want to "take the slack out of the bar" by pulling yourself into the bar as much as you can without the bar breaking off the floor.

This will create maximal stiffness and tension between you, the barbell, and the floor. Creating this "wedge" will make you stronger and safer.

As you pull yourself into the bar, open the toes, knees, and hips and create maximum tension.

When you are in this position, you are ready to begin the sumo deadlift.

Step 2 – The Sumo Deadlift

It's very important to not pick the weight off the floor. This is a common mistake that a lot of people make.

Instead, think about pushing the floor away from you. You want to do this in two ways. You will push the ground/floor away from you straight down, but you also need to "spread the floor." The sumo deadlift is very much a combination of pushing down and also pushing out.

Once you start pushing the floor away, keep maximum upper body tension. Once the bar breaks off the floor, the hips and shoulders should both rise at the same time.

As the bar starts to move off the floor, be sure to keep it as close to the body as possible. First it will be the shins, and then, as it crosses the knees, it will be close to the thighs.

When the barbell starts to move and is close to the body, once it passes the knees think about squeezing your quads hard and locking your knees. Note that locking your knees is not the same as hyperextending the knees.

As the bar passes the knees, squeeze your quads and then try to lock your knees. Once you do this then you want to immediately squeeze your glutes as hard as possible. While doing this you want to try to have the mass of your upper body "fall back," creating a counterbalance.

At the top of the sumo deadlift, you want to have knees locked, quads tight, hips locked, and shoulders in neutral position while standing erect and having full control of the barbell.

Step 3 – Lowering the Sumo Deadlift

It is very important that you reverse the motion of the sumo deadlift on the way down. This is where a lot of people make mistakes, and it's also where a lot of people get hurt during the deadlift.

Be sure that as you lower the bar you push the hips back first (hip hinge from the top down), and do not bend through the lower back. This is a very common error and can lead to back pain or injury.

Maintain upper body tension while keeping your core/trunk braced. Push the hips back and keep the bar close to your body as you lower the bar back to the floor.

Coach Rob's Tip:

A great way to improve and even master a technique is to move slowly. To learn the proper movement pattern and technique, start by moving very slowly with low weight. Then, over time, as the technique becomes sound, slowly start to improve your lifting speed.

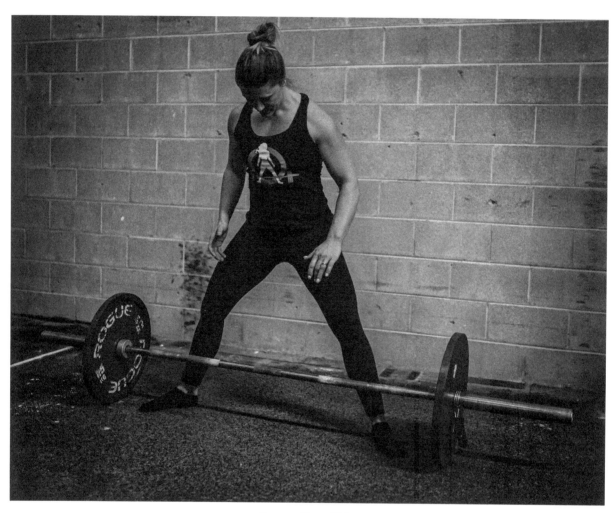

Sumo Deadlift

Four Types of Grips for Doing Deadlifts

1. Mixed Grip

The most common and effective grip for most people when deadlifting will be what's called a mixed grip.

With a mixed grip you will have one hand facing you and one hand facing away from you. If you raised your hands in front of your arms straight out ahead, you would have one palm facing up, and the other palm facing down.

There is no certain hand that should be on top or on bottom. Find what feels natural for you.

At first this grip may feel awkward and not normal; however, over time it should feel comfortable.

For the most part you can usually grip the most with this grip (while some may find the same with the hook grip).

You may also want to rotate your over and under hands to reduce the possibility of developing imbalances or asymmetries.

2. Hook Grip

A hook grip during a deadlift is where you have both palms facing toward you as you lift. Instead of "gripping" the barbell with your fingers, the main focus is to use your first and second fingers to grab your own thumb, thereby turning your hand into a hook.

You create a secure lock by holding and gripping your own thumb.

While this is painful at first, many people like this grip and it offers numerous benefits such as posture, positioning, reduction of injuries, and more.

This is a very difficult grip, however, if you have smaller hands and use a standard barbell with a diameter of 28 mm to 29 mm.

In powerlifting, there is only one size of barbell. In weightlifting, there is a women's barbell with a diameter of 25 mm.

3. Double Overhand Grip

Another common deadlift grip is known as double overhand. With this grip you grab the barbell with both palms facing toward you.

This is similar to a hook grip, but you are not gripping your own thumb.

This grip is usually a great way to learn the deadlift. As well, it's a great option for testing relative overall full body strength and grip strength.

Usually you will have the weakest grip with this grip, and again small hands will play a role.

However, I think it's great to focus on learning with double over grip and building double over grip strength on the deadlift.

4. Deadlift Grip Using Straps or Hooks

I often recommend that people use no grip tools when learning the deadlift. As well, I recommend using and trying all three normal grips when deadlifting.

There are times, however, when straps and hooks can have their place. Taking into consideration injuries, training goals, the inability to use chalk, and other things like this, straps and hooks can be great training tools for deadlifts.

I recommending using them as additional tools to improve your training or to help you work around some type of injury.

Coach Rob's Tip:

Focus on developing a strong deadlift grip strength. Try to avoid using gloves and straps. Build your hand and finger strength. This is important for deadlifting, and for you to get stronger. Your grip and hands may be a limiting factor at first, but you will adapt quickly. As well, when possible use chalk or liquid chalk.

Breathing and Bracing in the Deadlift

A great way to learn to breathe and brace for a deadlift can follow a simple principle. This principle is also great for beginners.

"If the bar is moving, you are not breathing."

Take a big breath into your core/trunk and hold it during the setup. Keep your air and tension as the bar is being lifted.

If you want to re-breathe, be sure to do so at the bottom of the lift when the bar is on the floor, or at the top of the lift.

If you re-breathe at the top of the sumo deadlift, be sure to keep your ribs down and maintain you brace as you "sip breath" or "straw breath." Picture yourself taking small sips of air or breathing through a straw. This will allow you to re-breathe while not allowing your ribs to rise or lose core and trunk tension/stiffness while you re-breathe at the top of the deadlift.

Head and Eye Position in the Sumo Deadlift

While there are countless trains of thought on this, my advice is very simple: play with your head and eye position and find what works and feels best for you.

If you want to look down, great.

If you want to look straight ahead, no problem.

If you want to look up toward the sky, that is fine as well.

I do not think head and eye position should be done in one certain way.

It's very individual to the lifter.

Do what feels natural, but be sure to every once in a while try something different and see how it feels.

As well, don't believe any of this nonsense about your glutes "shutting down" when you look down.

A general rule of thumb is try to keep most things in relatively "neutral" position, but in the end it's always best to find what works best for you as an individual.

Coach Rob's Tip:

The best head and eye position is the one that works for you. There is no right or wrong here. Practice and go with what may feel natural and strongest for you. When in doubt, a neutral neck and spine is always a good go-to.

#3 The Barbell Bench Press

The barbell bench press is a staple in powerlifting and just general overall strength training.

When it comes to women and the bench press, there are a few things you want to really focus on.

1. Mastery of Technique

Women generally lack the overall body size of men, and especially upper body size.

Therefore, it's of the utmost importance to focus on building a strong and solid foundation by relying on skill and technique.

Men can often "muscle" a lift because of their size, but women can rarely do this, especially in the bench press.

Be sure to build a strong technical foundation. This sets the stage for everything else.

2. Patience

After coaching thousands of women in all areas of fitness, strength, and lifting, I have observed many trends.

I see that women often lack the patience that is required for progress in strength training and lifting.

Patience applies even more to the barbell bench press because the amounts lifted on the bar are not as comparable for the squat and the deadlift.

Getting every extra pound or kilogram on the bar should always be the goal.

This is why with the bench press you need technique, patience, and a third important thing.

3. The Kaizen Principle

Kaizen: Sino-Japanese word for "improvement," referring to business activities that continuously improve.

What this basically means is the constant and never-ending improvement done over a very long period of time.

With bench press, you have to constantly work on technique, strength, accessory work, and much more.

Consistency with bench press plays a big role.

In summary, you have to make sure that you learn proper technique, rely on being patient with your training, and always try to get that 1% better every day and every workout, especially with the bench press.

Three Phases of the Bench Press

1. Setup
2. Take Out/Lift-off
3. The Press

The setup of the bench press is a very important factor for creating strength and safety. Like every lift, the setup is very important to get things perfect and tight before the start of a lift.

However, with the bench press I feel the setup is even more important because being in contact with the bench gives us more points of contact. Think of a bar on your back when the only contact area is the floor; this also goes for the deadlift. With the bench press, however, you are also in contact with the bench press rack.

I like to teach the bench press setup step by step, so here it is broken down.

Five Phases of the Bench Press Setup

Step 1 – Pinch and Tuck

Before you lie back onto the pad of the bench, pinch and tuck your shoulder blades. Think about doing the opposite of a shoulder shrug.

Step 2 – Set the Shoulders

After you pinch and tuck, you want to set the shoulders. There are many ways you can dig into the pad of the bench press by using the uprights, the bench, underhand gripping the bar, etc. You can also walk your feet on the bench to improve the arch and setup.

Once you set the shoulders and dig them into the bench, you want to then slightly push your body back toward your spotter. This will help you dig in even better. Think of your upper body and neck/head becoming like Velcro on the bench.

Step 3 – Set Your Grip

Setting the proper hand position and grip is critical in the bench press. You want to make sure that your hand position is equal and even. You can do this by using landmarks on the bar (the ring, the knurl, and the smooth).

There is no perfect grip or hand position, so it's important to play with different grips and widths. There are advantages and disadvantages to everyone.

When starting off, just make sure the grip is even on each side. Maintain a tight grip by squeezing the bar throughout the setup and the take out and during the whole lift.

Step 4 – Set the Feet

Setting the feet can be done in numerous ways. Some people will start with the feet on the bench and lower them one at a time. Some people will slide them up and back and dig them in. There are many ways to do this, and it takes practice and coaching experience.

The main factor here is setting the feet back and tight to create a base and lower body tension.

Step 5 – Get Ready to Receive the Barbell

Once everything is set from the shoulders, hands, and feet, you are then ready to take out the barbell or take a lift-off to begin the rep.

Coach Rob's Tip:

In the bench press, a strong setup should be tight and somewhat uncomfortable.

How to Use Leg and Hip Drive in the Bench Press

The bench press is primarily known as an upper body lift.

But if you want to be as strong as possible and bench as much weight as you can, it's important to learn to use full body strength and not just upper body strength.

Two big components of the bench press are known as leg drive and hip drive.

Leg Drive in the Bench Press

When you bench press, it's important to set a solid base and contact between you, the barbell, your body, the bench, and the floor.

As part of the setup process, during the bench press you want to focus on creating leg tension aka leg drive.

Pull your feet up and back toward your opposite shoulders. Try to dig your feet hard into the ground, creating a post.

Some lifters will set their toes; some will set their full foot. This is dictated by many factors such as leg length, training goals, competition rules, and much more.

Once your feet are set, focus on squeezing your legs and pushing the ground away. Think of trying to drive your body back toward your spotter. As you do this, keep pulling your shoulder blades back and down. This will encourage you to drive your chest up.

The more you focus on pushing the floor away from you and driving your body and force back toward your spotter, the more leg drive you will create.

Hip Drive in the Bench Press

With hip drive, the focus will be on the hip musculature of the body (along with the legs). The muscles of the hips can contribute significantly to improving bench press strength and lower body tension.

Go through your same setup process. As you set the shoulders, feet, and hands, you want to then begin focusing on creating tension in the hip area.

When creating hip drive, focus on contracting the glutes forcefully. Squeeze your glutes hard and think about driving your hips back toward your spotter.

Often people focus on pushing the hips toward the sky. This is not as effective, and it can also lead to a common failure in the bench press of having the glutes come off the bench. The glutes should maintain contact with the bench and "hover" the bench, touching ever so slightly.

A great way to picture this is by pretending that the bottom half of the bench press pad is non-existent. If there were no place for you to rest your glutes and lower body, how would you bench press?

This idea should be applied to the bench press when creating hip drive. Squeeze the glutes hard, drive them back toward your spotter, and just maintain a slight bit of contact with the bench.

Coach Rob's Tip:

In order for women to have a strong bench press, it's important to use your whole body, not just your upper body.

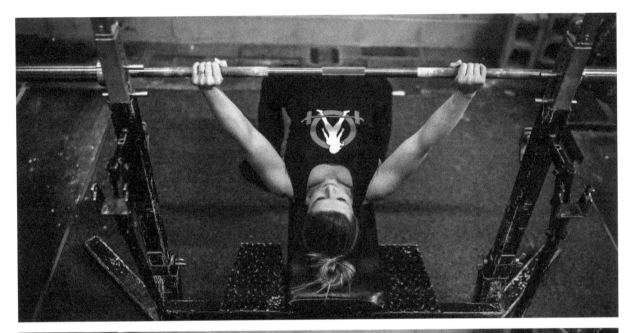

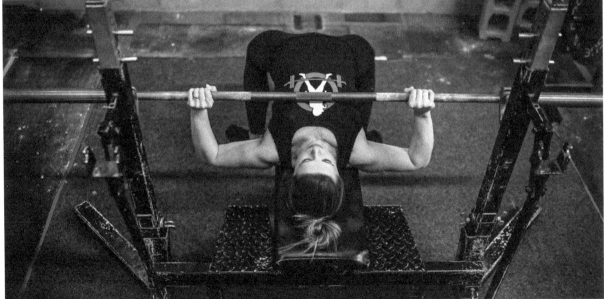

Barbell Bench Press

#4 The Barbell Overhead Press

The overhead barbell press is one of the best full body strength exercises that you can do.

When done properly, it's not just an upper body exercise; it's a full body exercise working everything. While it does have an upper body strength and muscle focus, the OH Press is a full body lift/exercise.

The OH press works the muscles of the shoulders, upper back, triceps, core, glutes, lower back, legs, and more.

How to Overhead Press:

Stand with the bar on your front shoulders and your hands next to your shoulders.

Press the bar over your head until it's balanced over your shoulders and midfoot.

Lock your elbows at the top.

Hold the bar for a second at the top. Then lower it back to your front shoulders and repeat. Don't use your legs; keep them straight.

Tip: To avoid shoulder pain, overhead press with a narrow grip so you don't flare your elbows. Then shrug your shoulders at the top. Press the bar over your head, lock your elbows, and shrug your shoulders toward the ceiling. This engages your traps and prevents shoulder impingement.

Coach Rob's Tip:

The overhead press is one of the best full body exercises.
It is also one of the most mentally satisfying exercises.
Putting weight overhead is a very powerful feeling.

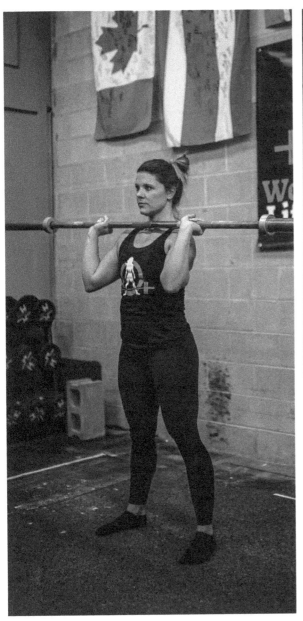 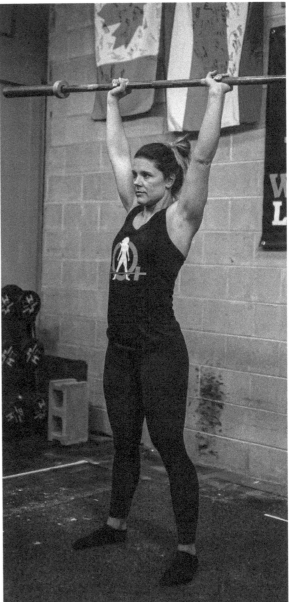

Barbell OH Press

#5 – The Barbell Lunge (Forward and Backward)

The barbell lunge is a single-leg strength exercise that works the quads, glutes, and hamstrings. This exercise will also improve hip mobility, core stability, and muscular balance on both sides of the body.

How to do a Forward Barbell Lunge

Set up a barbell on a rack at just below shoulder level.

Step under the bar, placing the back of your shoulders under it. Do not rest the bar on your neck.

Grip the bar using an overhand grip with your elbows bent to 90 degrees or slightly more. Less of an angle means your hands are too close together. This can cause instability of balance.

Lift the barbell clear of the rack by pushing with your legs while straightening your torso.

Step away from the rack.

Step forward with your right leg and squat down through your hips. Keep your back straight and be careful to maintain your balance. Inhale as you lower yourself.

Continue lowering your body until your left knee is nearly touching the floor.

Return to the start position by pushing through your heels, exhaling as you do so. Complete all the repetitions for one leg before switching.

Forward Lunge versus Reverse Lunge

The reverse lunge offers some variety and benefits when compared to a forward lunge. It is generally a bit more forgiving on the knee joint. As well, it has a larger focus on the glutes and hips versus the forward lunge which is more quad focused.

How to do a Barbell Reverse Lunge

Stand in a shoulder-width stance with a loaded barbell resting across your upper back. With palms facing outward, pull the bar down while squeezing your shoulder blades together for stability.

Push your chest out and take a large step backward, lowering your rear knee toward the ground while keeping your front shin as vertical as possible. Pause, and then push yourself back to the starting position by driving through the front heel and bringing your feet to meet each other.

CHAPTER 7

THE KETTLEBELL

A Personal Story About Kettlebells

I will be honest with you.

I used to think that the kettlebell was a farce of a training tool.

It was something that "looked cool" but had no real training benefits for athletes or for improving strength.

Boy, I was wrong.

Very wrong.

Enter the kettlebell.

Back in 2013, I was invited to attend a "StrongFirst" SFG certification by my friend and mentor Dan John.

I had very little to no knowledge or training with the kettlebell.

However, I decided a trip to Utah to learn from Dan John and Pavel had to be a great experience, so I decided to go (and thank you again, Coach Dan John).

I attended the StrongFirst SFG three-day certification in Utah and my life was changed in many ways physically and mentally.

One of the biggest changes was my knowledge and understanding of HOW to use the kettlebell.

I highly encourage you to read and learn from Coach Dan John and Coach Pavel Tsatsouline.

Thank you to my friend Coach Dan John for the opportunity and experience. The StrongFirst SFG Certification with him and Pavel in Utah was a life-changing experience.

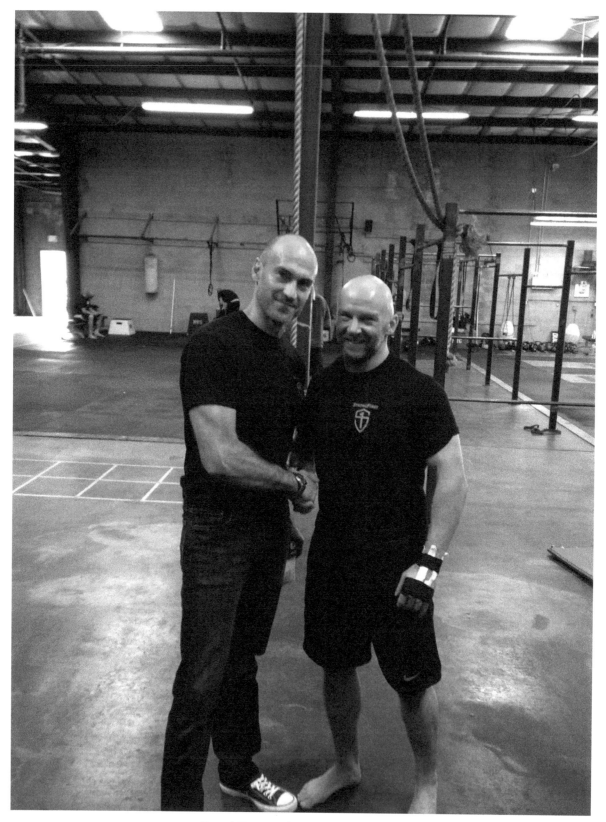

Pavel Tsatsouline & Coach Rob

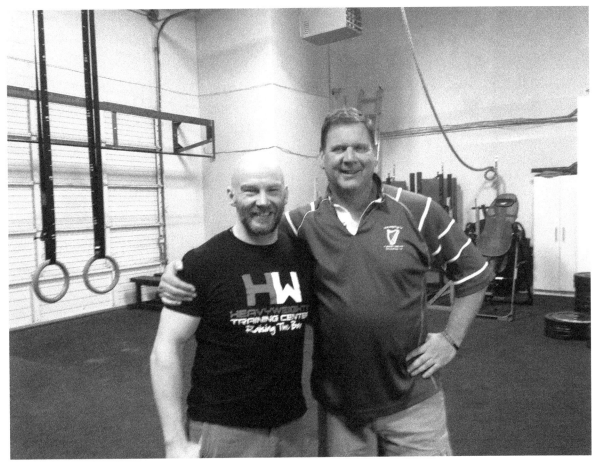

Dan John & Coach Rob

Kettlebells for Beginners: The Basics

The unique shape and uneven weight of the kettlebell make it a very effective functional training tool. You can take advantage of its structure to have fun with dynamic and ballistic movements that may not be possible or safe with other equipment like barbells or dumbbells.

The Anatomy of a Kettlebell

While there are many different types, styles, and even colours of kettlebells, they all within reason share the same basic anatomy.

1. **Handle:** The top part of the handle is commonly used to control movement.
2. **Corners:** The curved portion on each side of the handle starts to turn down toward the bell.

3. **Horns:** The two connection points are where each side of the handle meets the bell.
4. **Window:** This is the opening between the handle and the bell. Windows can be different sizes depending on the kettlebell style and manufacturer.
5. **Bell:** The bell is the centre of mass on the kettlebell. The bell is typically spherical.
6. **Base:** The flat portion at the bottom of the bell allows it to stand upright.

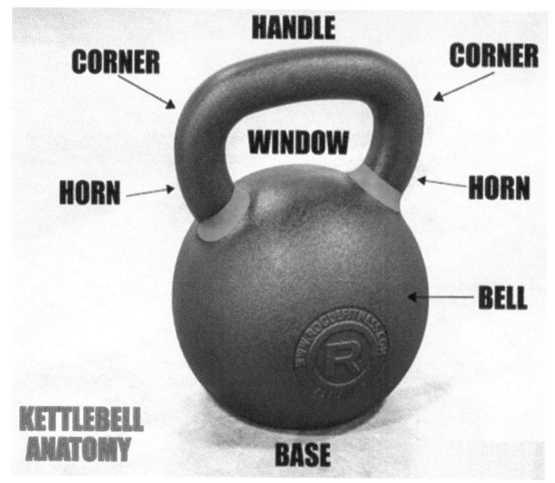

Kettlebell Anatomy

There are two main types of kettlebell.

- **Competition-style kettlebells** are made of steel and are all the same size regardless of their weight.

- **Classic kettlebells** are made of cast iron, and the size of the bell increases as its weight increases. Classic kettlebells also range in handle sizes, and the variety of handle thicknesses helps to work the grip.

CHAPTER 8

TOP FIVE KETTLEBELL EXERCISES

Top Five Kettlebell Exercises

1. Kettlebell Deadlift

2. Kettlebell Swing

3. Kettlebell Goblet Squat

4. Kettlebell Snatch

5. Kettlebell Get Up

The Kettlebell Deadlift

The kettlebell deadlift is a hip-hinge-based primary exercise used to develop full body strength with a major focus on the posterior chain.

I like to teach the KB deadlift in three steps.

1. Setup

2. Deadlift

3. Lowering

1. Kettlebell Deadlift – The Setup

It is recommended if possible, to deadlift in bare feet or a shoe with no padding or heel elevation when possible.

Step up to the kettlebell with the bell between your feet. Have the bell anywhere between your heels and midfoot. Try to avoid having it go toward your toes.

Set a tripod with your feet with the weight balanced evenly over your heel, big toe, and pinky toe.

Take a breath into your abdomen and brace your core/trunk.

Sit your hips back and keep your hips high. Continue to push your hips back while trying to maintain a vertical shin. Push your hips back into a high hip hinge position.

Have your arms go straight down as you continue to hinge. Keep your arms packed to your sides and close off your armpits; this will engage your lats.

Keep sitting your hips back, slightly bend your knees (soft knees), and slowly reach for the kettlebell. Once you reach the kettlebell, grip it tightly and pull yourself into the kettlebell to create a slight wedge between you, the kettlebell, and the floor.

Keep your eyes slightly down on the horizon.

2. Kettlebell Deadlift – The Lift

Once you have lowered properly in a hip hinge position and grabbed the bell, you are now ready to perform the deadlift.

Don't think about picking the kettlebell off the floor. Instead, grip the bell tightly and think about pushing the floor away from you.

As you push the floor away, drive your hips forward with force and contract your glutes/hips, making the bar break off the floor.

Once the bell starts moving off the floor, continue the motion and squeeze your glutes and hips. Keep your shoulders back and down, and keep your core/ribs down.

To finish the kettlebell deadlift, stand tall with your shoulders back, chest up, ribs down, knees and hips locked, and eyes straight ahead or slightly on the horizon.

From here you can exhale and or re-breathe for the lowering and/or next rep.

3. Kettlebell Deadlift – The Lowering

An important but neglected aspect of the kettlebell deadlift is the lowering (eccentric).

To lower the bell correctly, reverse the movement from the top down.

First, breathe, brace into your core, and create core tension/stiffness throughout the body.

Next, sit the hips back into a hip hinge position and start to slightly bend the knees. Keep the kettlebell close to your legs and keep the bell tight with your lats staying packed in and down. Lower the bell down toward the centre of your feet while maintaining a neutral spine with your eyes on the horizon.

Lower the bell with perfect form until it is back to the floor.

Coach Rob's Tip:

Learn and master the hip hinge.
It's a critical movement for maximum
strength, power, and safety.

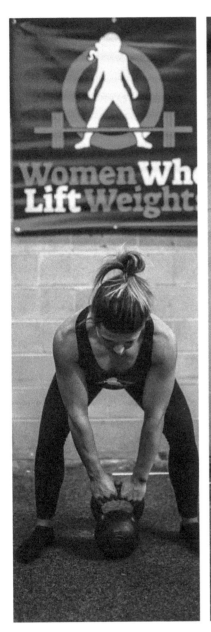
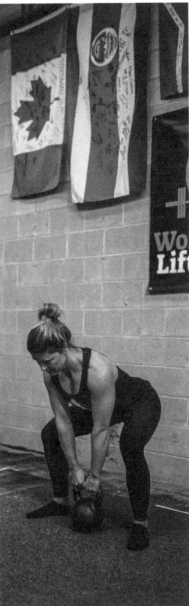
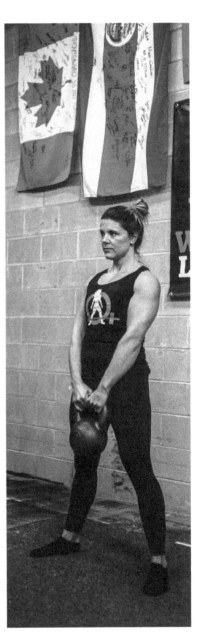

KB Dead lift

The Kettlebell Swing

How to do a Kettlebell Swing

I like to teach the KB swing in four steps.

1. The Setup
2. The Hike
3. The Swing
4. The Park

1. The Setup

Start with the kettlebell in front of you. As you look down, your feet and the kettlebell should make a triangle. Unlike the KB deadlift where you want the bell close to your midfoot or heels, with the swing you want to start the bell in front of you.

For the swing, it is recommended to do this barefoot or with shoes that have a flat sole with no padding in the soles or no lift in the heels.

Set your feet by gripping the floor and creating a tripod foot. Put weight evenly on the ball of the foot, the pinky toe, and the heel.

Once the feet are set, take a medium breath, breathe into your belly, and then brace your core.

The next step is to then push your hips back into a high hip hinge position. This is a very important part of the swing, so be sure to hinge and not bend through your lower back. Your spine should remain in neutral. As your hips go back, your chest can lean forward, almost like a deadlift position.

When you have loaded your hips with a strong hip hinge position, you can then reach for the bell. Reach first with one hand and then the other, grabbing the bell slightly to the outside. Do not grab the kettlebell too tightly. Once you have a grip on the bell, then tilt the horns of the bell toward you. Put the bell slightly on its side tilted toward you.

2. The Hike

When you are in a strong hip hinge position with your hands on the bell, you are loaded and ready to go.

From here you want to "hike" the kettlebell high toward your inner thighs. Think of a quarterback in football. The person in front of him is "hiking" the ball into his hands.

Hike the bell with force toward your inner thighs while maintaining your brace and a neutral spine. Once the bell goes between your inner thighs and behind you and you reach maximum distance, you are ready to fire the bell.

3. The Swing

As the bell goes back between your inner thighs, your hamstrings and glutes should be receiving all the tension. Almost like a bow and arrow, the hamstrings/hips are now loaded up and ready to fire.

Initiate the swing of the bell through a forceful hip contraction. As you squeeze your glutes and contract your quads, the bell should fly out in front of you.

Be sure to maintain core stiffness and upper body tension throughout the swing. You want to be tight, maintain control, and also move with speed.

The top part of the kettlebell swing while standing with the bell in front of you should be viewed as a standing "hard plank" with core braced, lats tight, legs tight, glutes tight, and the bell about sternum height with eyes straight ahead or slightly down on the horizon.

The bell should "float" momentarily. This is your rest moment. Enjoy it, as it's the only rest you get during the swing.

As the bell is floating, breathe out sharply through your mouth.

Once the bell reaches its apex, you want to initiate and pull the bell back down between your legs to the same place it was during the hike position.

Be sure to not just rely on letting gravity do its job; you want to try to "rip" the bell down with speed, power, and control.

Repeat this process for as many reps as desired or prescribed during the set.

4. The Park

Like lowering a barbell on the deadlift, it's very important to lower and return the kettlebell with proper form to where it started: slightly ahead of you on the floor.

For the last swing in your set, as the bell comes back between your legs you want to then control the swing. Instead of swinging toward the centre of the body again, you park the bell in front of you on the floor control. Ideally the bell wille be parked and returned to the same place you started your swing.

Coach Rob's Tip:

The kettlebell swing is a high-speed ballistic exercise.
Always respect the weight. Learning proper technique for
the swing is critical for effectiveness and safety.

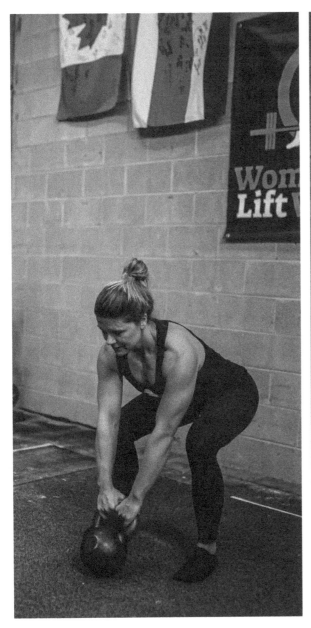
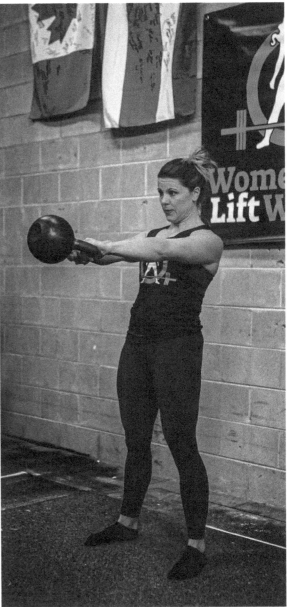

KB Swing

The Kettlebell Goblet Squat

The goblet squat is a great full-body exercise that builds muscle particularly in the legs, core, and glutes.

First of all, you want to find your squat stance. Have your feet about shoulder-width apart or a little bit wider. Point your toes straight ahead or have them pointed slightly out. Everyone's stance will be unique to them, so take some time to find the best squat stance for you.

Pick up the kettlebell off the floor with proper technique for safety.

Place the kettlebell in front of your chest about one inch in front of you. Try to keep your elbows tight, your core braced, and your lats tight.

Find your balance with your feet by gripping the floor. Make a tripod with the balls of your feet, your pinky toes, and your heels. Try to find a strong and stable balance position with your feet. This is also known as "rooting."

It's also a great idea to try to do the goblet squat barefoot or with flat shoes.

Once you are in a standing position and holding the kettlebell, you can begin the goblet squat.

The goblet squat starts with a lowering movement (eccentric).

Stand tall with your chest up and shoulders pick. Choose a spot ahead of you so that you have your eyes looking straight ahead or slightly down.

This is sometimes referred to as "eyes on the horizon."

Push your hips back and focus on sitting back. As you sit back, push the knees out slightly while being sure to keep them in line with your toes. As you bend your knees and sit back, try to keep tall with your chest up. One of the big benefits of the KB goblet squat is that having the weight in front of you will help you maintain this position.

Proceed to sit back, bend the knees, and drop your hips down.

As you are descending, breathe in through your nose.

Go as deep as you can with perfect posture and form.

Once you reach your depth, you want to change gears and reverse the motion and stand back up.

While keeping full body tension, push the floor away from you through the heels/midfoot. As you push the floor away, focus on squeezing your quads and then your hips as you stand back up to a standing neutral position.

As you are standing back up, breathe out through your mouth while maintaining your brace and keeping tension in your body.

Repeat each repetition with perfect form and technique.

Coach Rob's Tip

The goblet squat is one of the simplest and most effective squat variations you can do. It's a great variation to learn proper squat mechanics and body positioning.

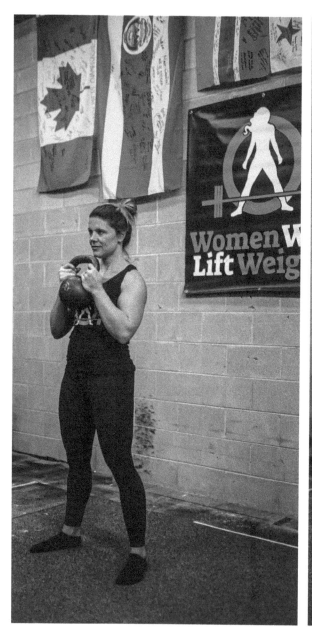 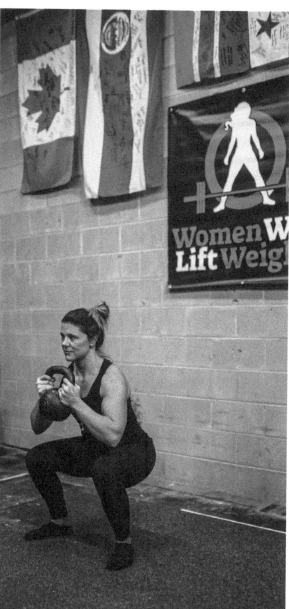

KB Goblet Squat

The Kettlebell Snatch

The kettlebell snatch is a movement where, after its initial hike, the kettlebell travels in a short upward arc with a bent arm and is stabilized overhead with a straight arm (lockout).

The kettlebell snatch is a great tool to build:

- Explosive total body strength
- A powerful grip
- A strong posterior chain (e.g., glutes, hamstrings)
- Solid core and upper body muscles
- Cardiovascular endurance and conditioning

While you can get these same benefits with one-handed kettlebell swings (especially heavier ones), snatching amplifies the muscle activation required to stabilize your body against two different motions: the forward pull of the kettlebell and the twisting created by the bell being off-centre.

While you may be very excited to delve into the kettlebell snatch, there are a few important things you'll need to master prior to snatching especially if it's your first time working with kettlebells.

One-Arm Swing

The one-arm swing trains similar stabilization as kettlebell snatching. It requires you to counter both the forward pull and the twisting motion of the kettlebell.

Being proficient in resisting these motions is necessary to eventually execute the snatch in a safe manner.

Overhead Lockout

Always make sure you can stabilize the bell in the overhead lockout position first. The lockout is a great kettlebell exercise on its own. Practicing overhead carries with a packed shoulder and a neutral wrist is a great way to build the shoulder stability that is needed to perform the kettlebell snatch.

To check your lockout, bring the bell up and into the overhead position with one arm. Carefully open your hand with your fingers up. The bell should be resting deep in your palm.

Note that you should always practice your lockout with overhead carries before moving to a heavier kettlebell for your snatch.

Grip During the Snatch

Training with kettlebells is a sure-fire way to develop hand calluses. To avoid unnecessary rips, practice having a nice hold without over-gripping. You can also use chalk or liquid chalk.

Start with the handle in the hook of your fingers. Work on bypassing your calluses on the way up. Have your hand open at the top of the snatch with the handle deep in your palm for the lockout.

Hike, Clean, and Press

Before you're ready to perform the snatch, make sure that you can hike, clean, and press a kettlebell. Safe execution here is essential to learning how to groove movements properly.

Coach Rob's Tip:

Don't grip the kettlebell too tightly; it will impact your technique and hurt your hands more. Unlike when doing barbell work where you want a tight grip, with KB training on swings, snatches, and cleans use a looser grip and allow the bell to move throughout your hands. As well when possible use chalk.

I like to teach the kettlebell snatch in four steps.

Step 1: The Mid Pull

The mid pull helps you "tame the arc" to keep the bell closer to the body than what you'd see in a one-arm swing, where the arm holding the kettlebell is fully extended at the shoulder. With this drill, keep your elbow close to your body to ensure that the kettlebell isn't casting out.

Start with your feet shoulder-width apart and the kettlebell in front of you. Hinge at the hips and hike the bell. Then, as you begin to snap your hips, pull the bell close to your body and keep your elbow attached to your rib cage.

Each mid pull finishes with the bell floating and your arms bent at a 90-degree angle. Then, you can quickly re-hike for the next rep.

Step 2: The Punch Thru

Also called a "horizontal snatch," do this with a very light bell. If you're a martial artist, it's time to get excited: this is literally a punch or strike (i.e., a very quick movement that you finish by locking out your elbow).

Start like the mid pull by moving into a hip hinge and hiking the bell back. Then, as you begin to snap your hips, pull the bell close to your body and keep your elbow attached to your ribcage.

Here's where the punch thru magic happens: the moment you finish your hip snap with a tension breath, punch your fist out, going from a bent elbow to a straight arm.

When you perform the punch thru, it's important to keep your shoulder packed, initiating the final movement from the elbow.

Step 3: The High Pull

While the high pull is an exercise on its own, it's also a fantastic drill to master before moving on to the snatch.

Go into your hip hinge position, hiking the bell back and forcefully snapping the hips as the kettlebell describes its arc. Instead of keeping your elbow glued to your side, let it move up and slightly back, as if you were trying to elbow someone standing behind you.

This movement is very quick, and the bell should float when the elbow is high by your ear. Then, you can quickly re-hike for the next rep.

Pay extra attention to your grip during the high pull. Use a hook grip and avoid squeezing the handle too tightly as this will restrict the natural movement of the bell.

Remember that the bell should be floating up thanks to the momentum created by the hip snap; you are never to muscle through a kettlebell movement like you would through the snatch.

Step 4: High Pull + Punch Thru = Snatch

Working with the progression of drills above, the hardstyle kettlebell snatch is essentially a combination of the high pull and the punch thru. You've made it to the finale!

How to do a Kettlebell Snatch

Start by hinging at the hips, and then hike the bell back. Snap the hips with a powerful tension breath as you keep the arc of the kettlebell close to your body. As the bell floats by your ear, punch the bell in an upward motion toward the ceiling.

This should bring you to a solid overhead position with the kettlebell sitting softly on your strong, straight wrist.

Pause momentarily, re-hike, and repeat.

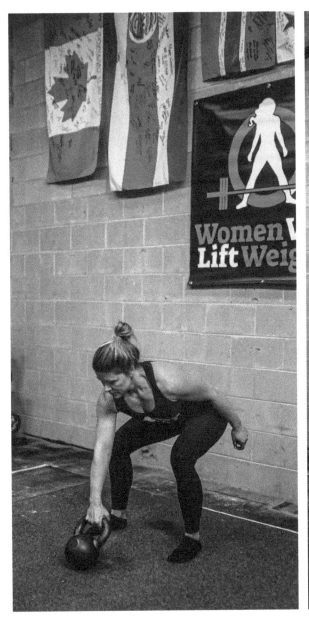
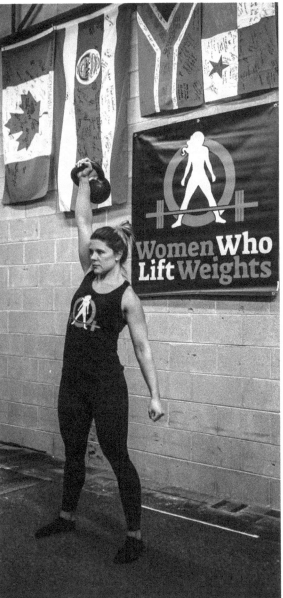

KB Snatch

The Kettlebell Get Up

If you have ever seen someone do a get up (also known as a "Turkish get up," you can see that when done properly it is a thing of beauty.

When done properly, it looks somewhat simple and easy, but don't be fooled. It is a very difficult and demanding exercise which requires technique, skill, strength, balance, coordination, and much more.

It's a great exercise for people of every age and fitness level; however, I think as we age this exercise becomes even more important.

The Turkish Get-up — Step-By-Step

Start on your back with the bell by your right side.

Roll into the fetal position and scoop your right hand through the handle, using the left hand for assistance.

Roll onto your back and press the bell to a full, locked-out, straight-arm position.

Place your left arm and leg straight on the floor, about 45 degrees away from midline (like a snow angel).

Next, place your right foot on the ground with your knee bent to 90 degrees. Leading with the chest, drive into the ground with all three non-loaded limbs until you have rolled up on your left forearm.

Keep both shoulders packed for the duration of the TGU and press through the palm of your hand until you left arm is straight (this is the "tall sit" position).

Press yourself slightly off the ground as you swoop your left heel toward your right foot, bringing your left knee toward your left hand. As you place your knee on the ground make sure your left hand, left knee, and left ankle form a straight line on the floor.

Hinge into the right hip, and then drive to full hip extension (as if finishing a swing) into a half-kneeling position.

Make a "windshield wiper" motion with the left leg so that both legs are now parallel in the bottom of a lunge position.

Dorsiflex the left foot (i.e., flex your foot so your toes are underneath you) and drive up to a standing position.

Take a large step back into the bottom of the lunge position, and "windshield wipe" the left leg.

Hinge at the hips and find the ground with your left hand (returning to that straight line with your left knee and left ankle).

Kick the left leg forward to the tall sit position, and then come down to your forearm.

Roll down onto your back and into the fetal position to return the bell to the floor.

Note that your eyes should be on your bell in all but two positions: the half-kneeling and standing.

Coach Rob's Tip:

Learn the get up with no weight at first other than your body weight. Practice each step. Stop at any sticking points. Practice that segment until you own it, and then proceed to the next. Once you learn how to do the get up with body weight, try doing it with a shoe or a sneaker in your hand for resistance and balance.

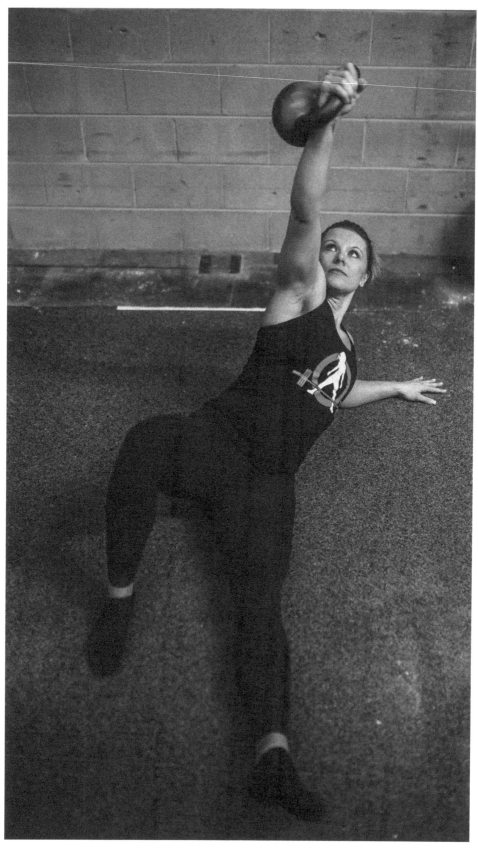

KB Get Up

CHAPTER 9

THE DUMBBELL

Introduction / Personal Story

My first introduction to lifting weights and strength training started with the dumbbell.

I was around 14 and I ventured into my brothers' room (I grew up with three older brothers and two older sisters).

Two of my brothers shared a tiny bedroom at the time, and in this tiny bedroom was one of those very old bench press setups with a basic slim barbell, a bench, and some old-school plastic and concrete dumbbells.

The weight bench and weights could barely fit in the tiny room, but they had their priorities in check.

My brothers liked to lift back in the day.

At the time I was a skateboarder (imagine me with long bangs and a full head of hair) and had no interest in lifting weights, although I was very much into martial arts.

I went into my brothers' room, grabbed some dumbbells, and started to lift.

I clearly had no idea what I was doing, nor did I know the impact that this would eventually have on my life.

My brother showed me a few little tips and tricks and how to do some exercises properly.

This would be my introduction to lifting.

A few years later my desire for strength and building muscle took a serious turn because of a girl... But I will leave that story for another day ☺.

The Dumbbell

I think that the dumbbell is one of the best tools you can use to build muscle, get stronger, lose fat, and improve performance.

Another huge benefit of dumbbell training is that it is somewhat more forgiving on the body than barbell training in many ways.

Dumbbells are unlimited in terms of the variety of exercises you can do, and once you add in things like tempo and other training variables, the sky is the limit.

I also feel that dumbbells are great for bodybuilding and building muscle in a different way than a barbell or a kettlebell can offer.

A low-cost investment of a few sets of dumbbells can lead to a full body workout with unlimited exercises and variations.

Dumbbells also complement the barbell and kettlebells nicely; you will see this when you get to chapter 13 with our programs.

CHAPTER 10

TOP FIVE DUMBBELL EXERCISES

Top Five Dumbbell Exercises

1. The Dumbbell Goblet Squat

2. The Dumbbell RDL (Romanian Deadlift)

3. The Dumbbell Lunge (Forward and Reverse)

4. The Dumbbell Bent Over Row

5. The Dumbbell Curl and Overhead Press

The Dumbbell Goblet Squat

The Dumbbell Goblet Squat is a great full-body exercise that builds muscle particularly in the legs, core, and glutes. It is very similar to using a kettlebell with a few small differences.

First of all, you want to find your squat stance. Have your feet about shoulder-width apart or a little bit wider. Point your toes straight ahead or have them pointed slightly out. Everyone's stance will be unique to them, so take some time to find the best squat stance for you.

Pick up the dumbbell off the floor using proper technique for safety.

Place the dumbbell in front of your chest about one inch in front of you. Try to keep your elbows tight, your core braced, and your lats tight. Use the palm of your hands to hold the dumbbell, almost like you are praying but with your fingers open and pulled back. Rest the dumbbell in the palms of your hands.

Find your balance with your feet by gripping the floor. Make a tripod with the balls of your feet, your pinky toes, and your heels. Try to find a strong and stable balance position with your feet. This is also known as "rooting."

It's also a great idea to try to do the goblet squat barefoot or with flat shoes.

Once you are in a standing position and holding the dumbbell, you can begin the goblet squat.

The goblet squat starts with a lowering movement (eccentric).

Stand tall with your chest up and shoulders pick. Choose a spot ahead of you so that you have your eyes looking straight ahead or slightly down.

This is sometimes referred to as "eyes on the horizon."

Push your hips back and focus on sitting back. As you sit back, push the knees out slightly, while being sure to keep them in line with your toes. As you bend your knees and sit back, try to keep tall with your chest up. One of the big benefits of the KB goblet squat is that it will help you maintain this position where you have the weight in front of you.

Proceed to sit back, bend the knees, and drop your hips down.

As you are descending, breathe in through your nose.

Go as deep as you can with perfect posture and form.

Once you reach your depth, you want to change gears, reverse the motion, and stand back up.

While keeping full body tension, push the floor away from you through the heels/midfoot. As you push the floor away, focus on squeezing your quads and then your hips. Stand back up to a neutral position.

As you are standing back up breath out through your mouth while maintain your brace and keeping your tension in your body.

Repeat each repetition with perfect form and technique.

Coach Rob's Tip:

*When doing heavy dumbbell goblet squats,
I recommend trying to pick up the weight off something
that is about chest height instead of picking the weight
up off the floor. A box or stool is perfect.*

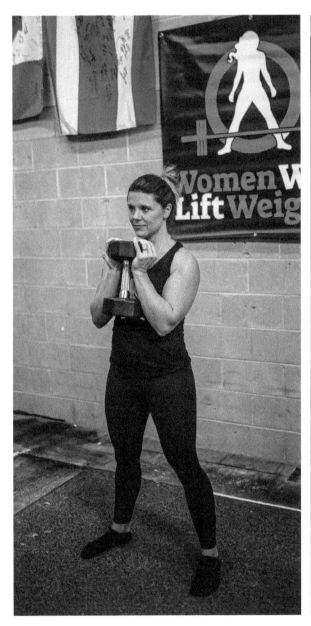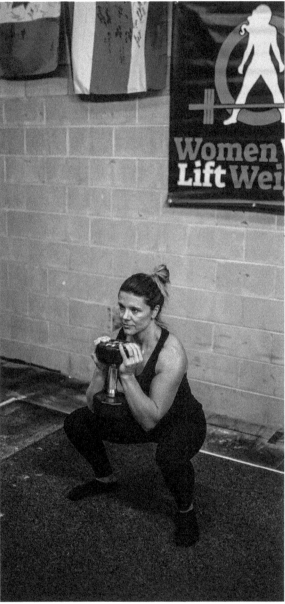

DB Goblet Squat

The Dumbbell RDL (Romanian Deadlift)

The dumbbell Romanian deadlift, also known as the dumbbell RDL, is an essential exercise for building strength in your legs and lower back. Not only will this exercise boost your lower body strength, it will help you develop proper form on other exercises as well.

The dumbbell Romanian deadlift works your hamstrings, glutes, and lower back.

How to do the Dumbbell Romanian RDL

Assume a standing position with your feet shoulder-width apart and hold the dumbbells with your palms facing inward.

Take a breath into your belly, brace your core, bring your shoulder blades together, and keep your chest held high.

With a slight bend in your knees (soft knees), perform a hip hinge at the waist with a straight back and lower the weights toward the ground.

You should feel a deep stretch in your hamstrings as your hips move backwards. Try to think about pushing your hips back and letting your chest come forward.

Try to push the weight toward the back of your midfoot and heel.

Once you reach the bottom of the rep and have achieved tension in the posterior change, reverse and start to come back to a standing position.

As you do, think about squeezing your glutes. Maintain core stiffness throughout the rep.

I prefer to breathe at the top and not breathe when the DBs are moving. You can breathe during reps for lighter weights, but when using heavy weights, be sure to breathe, brace, and hold tension similar to doing a barbell deadlift.

Coach Rob's Tip:

For even better results try to slightly elevate your toes.
You can use a 2.5 lb or 5 lb plate, or even the
handle of a kettlebell for this.

The Dumbbell Lunge (Forward and Reverse)

The dumbbell lunge is a single-leg strength exercise that increases strength in the quads, hamstrings, and glutes. The exercise also improves core stability and develops lower body strength.

Dumbbell Forward Lunge

Stand up straight with a dumbbell in each hand. Position your arms at your sides. Palms should face the thighs (hammer grip). Feet should be a little less than shoulder-width apart.

Take a step forward with either leg, bending at the knee until the front thigh approaches parallel to the ground, landing on the heel.

Inhale as you go down.

The rear leg is bent at the knee and balanced on the toes. For the leg you step forward with, don't let the knee go past the tip of the toes.

Step back to your standing starting position while exhaling.

Repeat the motion with the other leg.

Dumbbell Reverse Lunge

The dumbbell reverse lunge is a single-leg strength exercise that targets the glutes, hamstrings, and quads. The exercise also improves stability and balance on both sides of the body.

While forward and reverse lunges both work the glutes, legs, and abs, each emphasizes different leg muscles. Reverse lunges target more the hamstrings (back of thighs) and glute max (your meatiest glute muscle), whereas forward lunges focus more on the quads (front of thighs).

Another benefit is that for many people with knee pain, the reverse DB lunge is a more joint-friendly lunge.

Start by standing tall with feet hip-width apart. Grip dumbbells and hold at the side of your body. Step back one leg at a time, maintaining hip width. Ensure front knee travels slightly forward of toes and hamstring comes to touch calf muscle.

Maintain upright posture and strong torso whilst driving back up.

The Dumbbell Bent Over Row

I chose the dumbbell bent over row as a top five exercise for a few reasons. One of them is that it's a great "bang for your buck" exercise, hitting numerous things at once.

With the DB bent over row you can work a static hip hinge position, hitting the posterior chain along with targeting the muscles of the back such as the lats, the spinal erectors, and the biceps.

From a standing position perform a hip hinge RDL, putting the emphasis on the posterior chain and not the lower back.

From here, row the dumbbells toward the floor while trying to stretch through the lats. Maintain a neutral spine and don't round your upper back.

As the DBs descend away from you, have them stay close to the body. At the end of the rep, have the DBs go ahead from you slightly. This will increase the tension and stretch on the lats.

Once your arms reach full extension, proceed to row your arms to your side. It's important here to focus on stretching and contracting the muscles.

Coach Rob's Tip:

DB rows are all about working the muscles.
Choose a load that you can handle. Another great option
is using tempo work and slowing things down. Be sure to
stretch and squeeze your lats during this exercise.

The Standing Dumbbell Curl and Press

The DB curl and press is one of the most simple and effective upper body exercises.

As well, I recommend this exercise to be done standing with feet shoulder-width apart or with a staggered split stance.

Muscles worked during the standing curl and press include the biceps, the shoulders, the core, the glutes, and more.

How to do a Standing DB Curl and Press

Start with your feet shoulder-width apart. Place your arms by your sides with your palms facing out.

Bend your forearms until your hands — or weights — touch your shoulders. Make sure your elbows are kept firmly by your sides for this movement.

Keeping your arms here, rotate your palms so that they're facing forward.

Push your arms over your head until both arms are extended straight above your body, keeping your core activated and straight. Lower your shoulders away from your ears.

Slowly lower your arms with your palms still facing forward until your palms are parallel with your shoulders.

Turn your palms toward you and slowly lower your triceps, with your elbows firmly next to your torso, until your arms are completely hanging by your sides.

Coach Rob's Tip:

While this exercise can be done sitting on a bench, it will target the upper body more by taking out the lower body. I recommend doing this exercise from a standing position so that it will challenge the whole body.

CHAPTER 11

HOW TO DO A PROPER WARM-UP AND COOL-DOWN FOR A STRENGTH-TRAINING WORKOUT

I'm going to share with you a little secret. One of the biggest mistakes that most people make when training is neglecting the warm-up and the cool-down.

The warm-up especially is a very important part of your workout and your training.

What is a warm-up and why would this benefit your training and results?

Let's discuss this in a bit more detail.

What is a "Warm-up?"

A "warm-up" is essentially taking some time to get your body (and your mind) ready for the workout.

We are all busy in life, but a warm-up should only take between five and fifteen minutes. It doesn't have to take long. After a while, you should be able to do a quick but effective warm-up before you start your strength-training sessions.

A Warm-up Should Accomplish three Major Things:

1. Increase body temperature;
2. Get your body ready to train and perform; and
3. Reduce muscle soreness and lessen your risk of injury.

How to Warm Up for a Strength-training Workout

Let's look over a sample warm-up and why we would do what we do.

1. Get Body Temperature Up

A simple thing you can do here is some type of light aerobic- or calisthenic-type workout.

Calisthenics are exercises that don't rely on anything but a person's own body weight.

The goal here is pretty simple: get your core body temperature up and sweat a little.

You could do a few minutes on a bike or machine, light skipping, or body weight movements like light jogging or jumping jacks, etc.

You can do anything to get the body warm and ready for the workout ahead.

This should only take about five minutes.

2. Dynamic Mobility + Muscle Activation

In simple terms, a dynamic warm-up is "moving while you stretch" or stretching through a joint's full range of motion and preparing muscles for more intense exercise to come. A dynamic warm-up promotes blood flow, helps prevent injury and muscle soreness, as well as helps improve overall performance.

I always try to think about getting the "ball and socket" joints warm and moving. The ball and socket joints of the body are the hip and the shoulder. We want blood flow and movement in these joints to get us ready for strength training.

Along with dynamic mobility, you also want to "wake up" some of the muscles or movements that you are going to do.

This is known as "muscle activation."

Let's say I am going to do a squat workout. There are certain areas and muscles that I need to focus on.

These areas are:

- Warming up and improving mobility of the hip joint
- Warming up the muscles of the lower body (quads, glutes, hamstrings)
- Adding in some core work as the core plays a big role in stabilizing the squat

Here is a sample six-exercise mobility/stability warm-up for squats:

1. Kettlebell prying goblet squats — three sets of ten
2. Hip rockers — three sets of ten
3. Shoulder rotations — tens sets of front and back
4. Dynamic hamstring stretch — three sets of ten
5. "Hard plank" — ten seconds three times
6. Glute bridge – 3 sets of 10

3. Pay Attention to Things that are Important to You

Find exercises and movements that are important to you as an individual.

For this we need to consider such things as:

- Age
- Previous injuries
- Genetic limitations
- Climate (do you live somewhere cold or somewhere warm?)
- The movement you are warming up for (for example a bench warm-up is similar but different from a squat or deadlift warm-up)
- Muscle soreness and fatigue

It's important that you try to get "in tune" with your body. This improves with time and training.

The best warm-up you can do is one that suits your body and your training needs by taking into consideration the above three main factors.

What About Static Stretching?

Static stretches are those in which you stand, sit, or lie still and hold a single position for a period of time of approximately 30 to 60 seconds.

A little tip that is important: don't do static stretching before you train. Static stretching can reduce strength and performance.

Static stretching should only be done after training.

What is a "Cool-down?"

Cooling down is an easy exercise, done after a more intense activity, to allow the body to gradually transition to a resting or near-resting state. Depending on the intensity of the exercise, cooling down can involve a slow jog or walk. With lower intensities, stretching can be used.

You could also add in some soft tissue work like foam rolling along with some relaxation and deep-breathing exercises.

Benefits of a Cool-down

Cooling down allows your body temperature, blood pressure, and heart rate to return to their normal levels. Stretching your muscles while they're still warm can help to reduce lactic acid buildup, thereby reducing your chance of muscle cramps and stiffness.

Often when we lift weights our CNS (Central Nervous System) gets very aroused and excited. As you try to relax after an intense lifting session, it can be very difficult to unwind. A cool-down can help with this.

How to Cool Down After a Strength-training Workout

Personally, I find that a five- to ten-minute cool-down after a training session goes a long way.

After a cool-down you should feel calm and restored.

Coach Rob's Tip:

Before training, take five to ten minutes.
Focus on improving core temperature, adding in some dynamic mobility and muscle activation.
After your training, focus on a mixture of light cardio, static stretching, and soft tissue work along with deep breathing exercises to relax the mind and body.

CHAPTER 12

STRENGTH-TRAINING PROGRAMS

Now that you have the basic tools and exercises, you can start to put the pieces together.

A training tool is nothing without use and knowledge.

The barbell, kettlebell, and dumbbell each bring their own elements to training and program design.

The better your knowledge and understanding of each training tool, the better the results you can achieve.

A Note on Minimalism and Basics in Training

We live in a world of abundance in life and at the gym.

There are thousands of training machines and pieces of equipment, and there is no lack of knowledge and information at our fingertips with the internet.

However, when it comes to strength training, more is not always better; if anything, more gets in the way of progress.

It's easy to always be looking for new or for more: a new training tool, a new exercise, a new workout program, a new machine, a new watch to track your progress.

We all suffer from shiny object syndrome.

It's important to understand that strength training isn't about more. It's about using what you have and knowing how to make the most of what you have.

Without question, having 100 training tools to use can give you more variety with exercises and programming, but come the end of the day, getting stronger is not about how many things you have. It's about putting in the work and paying your dues.

There is no substitute for hard work.

There is no substitute for The Iron.

Stop looking around for the next best thing, the newest gadget, or the shiniest object.

Instead, invest your time and energy into understanding how to use the basic strength-training tools such as the barbell, the kettlebell, and dumbbells.

While variety is great and sometimes needed, there is no substitute for a good daily dose of The Iron.

The Programs

In these programs, I offer you a very basic, simple, and minimalist approach to training.

The goal is to not complicate, but rather to simplify.

Each program is based on using each tool on its own, and then also combining tools together.

Think of it like compound interest but for strength training.

However, you don't need to add more tools until you have a solid grasp of the fundamentals in terms of exercises and movement.

Each training tool brings its own benefits and drawbacks. Not every exercise will be the right exercise for everyone.

We have to consider the training tool, the person, the history of the person, injuries, knowledge of the how to use each training tool, and much more.

There are thousands of variations of exercises when you combine all three tools, but remember that the goal is simplicity, not complexity.

Come the end of the day, it doesn't matter if your program can be written on a napkin or if you need a fancy app to contain it. Either way, you have to do the work.

The True Focus of Strength Training

It's important to note that the focus of strength training should be to improve strength.

Women oftentimes have a tendency to search for fatigue, not necessarily progress. Keep in mind there is a big difference between the two.

Proper strength training requires effort, patience, and time. Most women love to put in the work but often lack the patience and time needed.

With lifting and strength training you have to "pay time under the bar" as the saying goes. No matter how hard you work, you have to be patient and give things time

Oftentimes they will believe the old myths that "more is better" or "do more in less time."

While there are times that these sayings can hold truth, when it comes to lifting weights and strength training, this is not the case.

You must prioritize rest during your workout, and you must prioritize rest after your workout.

The goal of strength training is to get better, not get tired.

> *"Anyone can make you tired, not anyone can make you better."*
> *—Martin Rooney, Training For Warriors*

The Body is a System

Think of each workout as a full body workout first and foremost.

We may add in some body part training with barbell and dumbbell movements, but our main focus is training the body as a system, not just a bunch of individual body parts.

There is nothing wrong with the typical bodybuilding-style workouts that are commonly referred to as "body part split" training; however, when it comes to strength, it's important to first view the body as a complete system that works in synergy to produce strength and power.

It's important to note that these programs are not designed as "bodybuilding" programs. These basic strength-training programs are designed to get your body strong from head to toe, and to create full body strength and muscles that perform, not just look good. The by-product, however, will be overall strength and muscles that look amazing and perform.

I think it's important to develop a good base of strength-training basics and full body strength, and then to accessorize with body part movements to improve specific areas for building more muscle or improving areas of strength.

A strong foundation of lifting technique and full body strength needs to be a priority.

Program Design

Each program will be strength-focused with some variations.

These programs take a mixture of powerlifting basic barbell lifts and adding them in with "hard-style" kettlebell movements along with power-building dumbbell movements and exercises.

Rest Time

For simplicity's sake, in these programs I suggest an average amount of time needed between sets.

Each athlete will have different rest times based on goals, strength levels, recovery levels, age, stress, lifestyle, etc.

We could make this as complicated as we want, but let's not.

For simplicity's sake, consider the following three points when it comes to rest:

1. Rest as long as you need to before your next set.
2. Don't be tired in any way before your next set.
3. When in doubt, time your rest and, if possible, your heart rate.

Oftentimes women will think they are rested and good to go for the next set before they usually are.

This is especially true when it comes to heavy barbell lifts and strength training.

Rest Time For Lifting Heavy Weights

The heavier you go, the more rest time you need.

For example, a heavy set of barbell squats or deadlifts will require much more time for recovery compared to say a set of kettlebell goblet squats or deadlifts.

While both lifts can be demanding in their own way, the much larger amount of weight lifted on a compound barbell exercise will cause a bigger drain on the body/system from a recovery standpoint.

Basic barbell compound lifts and exercises have a far bigger demand on the CNS (central nervous system) than the demand of kettlebell or dumbbell exercises.

Be sure to allow enough rest time during your heavy lifting sessions.

Remember the goal is to get stronger and better, not to get tired.

The goal should be to maintain strength during your workout. If at any point you notice your strength dropping, this usually means a couple of things:

1. You didn't rest long enough.
2. You pushed too hard.
3. Your workout is too long and you are doing too much.
4. See #1, #2, or #3.

Rest Time Simplified

To increase Strength and Power as quickly as possible, the best rest period is 2 minutes to 10+ minutes between sets. This will be determined by the weight lifted, the intensity of the lift, the load of the lift and the experience of the lifter.

To increase Hypertrophy (muscle building) as quickly as possible, the best rest period is 30 to 90 seconds between sets.

To increase Muscular Endurance as quickly as possible, the best rest period is 30 seconds or less between sets.

Rest Time For Body Part Training and Accessory Lifts

When it comes to kettlebell and dumbbell exercises, we usually require less rest than we do from barbell compound lifts.

Each person will require different rest times based on many variables, but the principle should remain the same.

The goal is to not lift tired; the goal is to not get tired.

Even though kettlebell and dumbbells may require less rest time when compared to a barbell, it's still important to not neglect rest and recovery time.

Let's go back and review three basic principles for rest and recovery during training:

1. Rest as long as you need to before your next set.
2. Don't be tired in any way before your next set.
3. When in doubt, time your rest and, if possible, your heart rate.

Rest Time Simplified

To increase strength and power as quickly as possible, the best rest period is two to five minutes between sets.

To increase hypertrophy (muscle building) as quickly as possible, the best rest period is 30 to 90 seconds between sets.

To increase muscular endurance as quickly as possible, the best rest period is 30 seconds or less between sets.

How to Use As and Bs in these Programs

I learned how to write programs from many different coaches over my many years in training. I have been influenced by powerlifting programs and coaches, kettlebell coaches and programs, bodybuilding coaches and programs, and much more.

One person, however, who has played a huge role in how I write programs is Coach Charles Poliquin (aka The Strength Sensei).

Charles' programs would be based off a organized structure using A, B, C.

Let me explain.

Take a look at the following barbell workout:

A1. Barbell back squats — five sets of five reps (70%)

B1. Barbell bench press — five sets of eight reps

Rest one minute between sets.

B2. Barbell bent over rows — five sets of eight reps

C1. Barbell overhead press — three sets of eight reps

Rest one minute.

C2. Barbell RDL — three sets of eight reps

Rest one minute.

C3. Plank one minute.

For this workout, you would do all of the A exercises first. We only have one exercise in A for this example. You will not do any movements or exercises in B or C until all of A is completed.

Once the A series is done, then you would move on to B.

With B, we have a combination of two exercises.

You would do the B1 variation first, followed by the B2 variation.

You would complete all B exercises before proceeding to C.

In this workout, C has three exercises.

You would start with C1, then C2, and then C3.

As you can see, C3 is a body weight exercise at the very end which is less demanding.

You would finish all C variations as prescribed in the program.

Barbell Only Workout — Four-day Split

Focus

Primary Focus – Strength Training
Secondary Focus – Muscular Hypertrophy

You can do your four days in whatever way is best for you.

Examples:

> Monday – Day 1
> Tuesday – Day 2
> Wednesday – Rest

Thursday – Day 3
Friday – Day 4
Saturday and Sunday off

Or

Monday – Day 1
Tuesday – Rest
Wednesday – Day 2
Thursday – Rest
Friday – Day 3
Saturday – Rest or Day 4
Sunday – Day 4 or Rest

The exercise is listed first followed by the number of sets and the number of reps in each set. Notes on rest period or the amount of weight to use may be added as well.

Run this program for four to eight weeks. Increase weights as needed to keep the training challenging.

However, do not max out; do not "grind" or go too hard.

This is a "building phase" program, not a "peaking program"

Please note that reps come first followed by sets.

This workout is designed if you have ONE barbell.

If you have access to another barbell, you can pair the exercises.

For example:

A1. Barbell squats

Rest three minutes.

A2. CG (close grip) bench press

Rest two minutes.

I would not pair more than two or three barbell exercises in a row if you are looking for strength.

Recommended Rest Time for Barbell Training

Please note that recovery and recovery time is of the utmost importance for barbell strength training.

General Rest Time Chart

Rest training can be broken down into three areas:

Light weights – (twelve to twenty reps) thirty to ninety seconds
Medium weights – (eight to twelve reps) two to five minutes
Medium heavy weights (five to eight reps) five to eight minutes
Heavy weights – (one to five reps) eight to twelve-plus minutes

The Workouts

Please note you can download all these programs in excel and .pdf by visiting our website here =>

www.WomenWholiftWeights.com/StrengthGuidePrograms/

The Workout — Barbell Only Strength

Four-day Strength-training Program

STRENGTH TRAINING PLAN #1   Barbell Only - Primary Strength & Hypertrophy Focus

Coach: Robert King

	Week 1			Week 2			Week 3			Week 4			Week 5			Week 6		
Day 1	SETS	WT	REPS	SETS	WT	REPS	SETS	WT	REPS	SETS	WT	REPS	SETS	WT	REPS	SETS	WT	REPS
A1. Barbell Back Squats	3	70.0%	5	4	70.0%	8	5	70.0%	5	3	75.0%	5	4	75.0%	5	5	80.0%	5
B1. Barbell CG Bench Press	3	60%	8	4	60.00%	8	5	60%	8	3	65%	8	4	65%	8	5	65%	8
B2. Barbell Bent Over Row	3		8	3		8	4		8	3		8	4		8	5		8
C1. Standing Barbell Push Press	3		8	4		8	5		8	3		10	4		10	5		10
D1. Barbell Hip Thursts	3		8	4		10	5		15	3		12	4		15	5		15
Day 2	SETS	WT	REPS	SETS	WT	REPS	SETS	WT	REPS	SETS	WT	REPS	SETS	WT	REPS	SETS	WT	REPS
A1. Bench Press	3	60%	8	3	65.00%	8	3	70%	8	4	60%	6	4	65%	6	5	75%	5
B2. RDL Romanian Deadlift	3		8	4		8	5		8	3		8	4		8	5		8
C1 Deadlifts (light)	3		5	4		5	5		5	3		8	4		8	5		8
D2. Front Squats	3		5	4		5	5		5	3		5	4		5	5		5
Day 3	SETS	WT	REPS	SETS	WT	REPS	SETS	WT	REPS	SETS	WT	REPS	SETS	WT	REPS	SETS	WT	REPS
Active Rest / Recovery Day Add foam rolling, mobility, Conditioning																		
Day 4	SETS	WT	REPS	SETS	WT	REPS	SETS	WT	REPS	SETS	WT	REPS	SETS	WT	REPS	SETS	WT	REPS
A1. Deadlifts	3	70%	5	4	70%%	5	5	70%	5	3	75%	5	4	75.00%	5	5	75.00%	5
B1. Barbell Bench w Pause	3	RPE 7	5	4	RPE 7	5	5	RPE 7	5	3	RPE 8	5	4	RPE 8	6	5	RPE 8	8
B2 Deadstop Barbell Row	3		8	4		8	5		8	3		10	4		10	5		10
D1. Barbell Hip Thursts	3		12	4		12	5		12	3		15	4		15	5		15
Day 5	SETS		REPS	SETS		REPS	SETS		REPS	SETS		REPS	SETS		REPS	SETS		REPS
A1. Barbell Military Press	3		8	4		8	5		8	3		10	4		10	5		10
B1. Barbell Walking Lunges	3		8	4		8	5		8	3		10	4		10	5		10
C1. Barbell Row	3		8	4		8	5		8	3		10	4		10	5		10
D1. Barbell Hip Thursts	3		8	4		8	5		8	3		10	4		10	5		10
Day 6 & 7	SETS	WT	REPS	SETS	WT	REPS	SETS	WT	REPS	SETS	WT	REPS	SETS	WT	REPS	SETS	WT	REPS
Rest/Active Recovery Day																		

Notes:

Women Who Lift Weights

Coach: Robert King

info@womenwholiftweights.com

Kettlebell Only Workout — Four-day Split

Focus

Primary Focus – Muscular Conditioning
Secondary Focus – Strength / Performance

You can do your five days in whatever way is best for you.

Examples:

Monday – Day 1
Tuesday – Day 2
Wednesday – Rest
Thursday – Day 3
Friday – Day 4
Saturday – Rest
Sunday – Rest

Or

Monday – Day 1
Tuesday – Day 2
Wednesday – Rest
Thursday – Rest
Friday – Day 3
Saturday – Day 4
Sunday – Rest

You can vary these days for whatever works best for you based on schedule, recovery, injuries, and life.

The exercise is listed first, and then the number of sets and the number of reps in each set. Notes on rest period or the amount of weight to use may be added as well.

Run this program for four to eight weeks. Increase weights as needed to keep the training challenging. You can also reduce the rest time as well.

The goal is to always perform all lifts with perfect form. Never sacrifice poor form to save time. Quality training and lifts always come first.

You may use the same kettlebell for all exercises. However, if possible have more than one bell as each exercise is demanding in its own way.

Barbell Only Full Body Strength & Hypertrophy

Kettlebell Only Full Body Strength & Conditioning

STRENGTH TRAINING PLAN #2

Coach: Robert King

Kettlebell Only - Conditioning & Full Body Strength Focus

Exercise	W1 SETS	W1 WT	W1 REPS	W2 SETS	W2 WT	W2 REPS	W3 SETS	W3 WT	W3 REPS	W4 SETS	W4 WT	W4 REPS	W5 SETS	W5 WT	W5 REPS	W6 SETS	W6 WT	W6 REPS
Day 1																		
A1. Kettlebell Goblet Squat	3		6	4		6	5		6	4		8	4		8	5		8
B1. Kettlebell Snatch	3		6	4		6	5		6	4		8	4		8	5		8
C1. Kettlebell Military Press	3		6	4		6	5		6	4		8	4		8	5		8
D1. Kettlebell Hip Thrusts	3		12	4		12	5		12	4		15	4		15	5		15
E1. Kettlebell Suit Case Carry (1 Arm)	3		30 Seconds Each Arm	3		35 Seconds Each Arm	3		40 Seconds Each Arm	3		45 Seconds Each Arm	3		55 Seconds Each Arm	3		60 Seconds Each Arm
Day 2																		
A1. Kettlebell Swing	3		10	4		10	5		10	3		12	4		12	5		12
B1. Kettlebell Push Press	3		8	4		8	5		8	3		10	4		10	5		10
C1. Kettlebell Goblet Squats (2 Second Pause)	3		5	4		5	5		5	3		8	4		8	5		8
D1. Kettlebell Hip Thrusts (2 Sec Pause)	3		12	4		12	4		12	4		15	4		15	5		15
E1. Kettlebell Farmers Walk (2 Arm)	3		30 Seconds Each Arm	3		35 Seconds Each Arm	3		40 Seconds Each Arm	3		45 Seconds Each Arm	3		55 Seconds Each Arm	3		60 Seconds Each Arm
Day 3																		
Rest/ Active Recovery																		
Day 4																		
A1. Kettlebell Goblet Squat Single Arm Rack	3		6	4		6	5		6	4		8	4		8	5		8
B1. Kettlebell Deadlifts (2 Second Pause)	3		6	4		6	5		6	4		8	4		8	5		8
C1. Kettlebell 1 Arm Row	3		6	4		6	5		6	4		8	4		8	5		8
D1. Kettlebell Snatch	3		8	4		8	5		8	3		10	4		10	5		10
E1. Kettlebell Suit Case Carry (1 Arm)	3		30 Seconds Each Arm	3		35 Seconds Each Arm	3		40 Seconds Each Arm	3		45 Seconds Each Arm	3		55 Seconds Each Arm	3		60 Seconds Each Arm
Day 5																		
A1. Kettlebell Swing	3		10	4		10	5		10	3		15	4		15	5		15
B1. Kettlebell Push Press	3		8	4		8	5		8	3		10	4		10	5		10
C1. Kettlebell Goblet Squats (2 Second Pause)	3		5	4		5	5		5	3		8	4		8	5		8
D1. Kettlebell Hip Thrusts (2 Sec Pause)	3		12	4		12	4		12	4		15	4		15	5		15
E1. Kettlebell Farmers Walk (2 Arm)	3		30 Seconds Each Arm	3		35 Seconds Each Arm	3		40 Seconds Each Arm	3		45 Seconds Each Arm	3		55 Seconds Each Arm	3		60 Seconds Each Arm
Day 6 & 7																		
Rest/Active Recovery Day																		

Notes:

Women Who Lift Weights

Coach: Robert King

info@womenwholiftweights.com

Dumbbell Only Workout

STRENGTH TRAINING PLAN #3

Dumbbell Only - Hypertrophy & Full Body Strength Focus

Coach: Robert King

Day 1	Week 1 SETS	Week 1 WT	Week 1 REPS	Week 2 SETS	Week 2 WT	Week 2 REPS	Week 3 SETS	Week 3 WT	Week 3 REPS	Week 4 SETS	Week 4 WT	Week 4 REPS	Week 5 SETS	Week 5 WT	Week 5 REPS	Week 6 SETS	Week 6 WT	Week 6 REPS
A1. Dumbbell Goblet Squat	3		6	4		6	5		6	4		8	4		8	5		8
A2. Dumbbell Snatch	3		6	4		6	5		6	4		8	4		8	5		8
A3. Dumbbell Military Press	3		6	4		6	5		6	4		8	4		8	5		8
A4. Dumbbell Hip Thrusts	3		12	4		12	5		12	4		15	4		15	5		15
A5. Dumbbell Suit Case Carry (1 Arm)	3		30 Seconds Each Arm	3		35 Seconds Each Arm	3		40 Seconds Each Arm	3		45 Seconds Each Arm	3		55 Seconds Each Arm	3		60 Seconds Each Arm

Day 2	SETS	WT	REPS	SETS	WT	REPS	SETS	WT	REPS	SETS	WT	REPS	SETS	WT	REPS	SETS	WT	REPS
A1. Dumbbell Swing	3		10	4		10	5		10	3		12	4		12	5		12
A2. Dumbbell Push Press	3		8	4		8	5		8	3		10	4		10	5		10
A3. Dumbbell Goblet Squats (2 Second Pause)	3		5	4		5	5		5	4		8	4		8	5		8
A4. Dumbbell Hip Thrusts (2 Sec Pause)	3		12	4		12	5		12	4		15	4		15	5		15
A5. Dumbbell Farmers Walk (2 Arm)	3		30 Seconds Each Arm	3		35 Seconds Each Arm	3		40 Seconds Each Arm	3		45 Seconds Each Arm	3		55 Seconds Each Arm	3		60 Seconds Each Arm

Day 3 Rest/ Active Recovery

Day 4	SETS	WT	REPS	SETS	WT	REPS	SETS	WT	REPS	SETS	WT	REPS	SETS	WT	REPS	SETS	WT	REPS
A1. Dumbbell Goblet Squat Single Arm Rack	3		10	4		10	5		10	4		8	4		8	5		8
A2. Dumbbell Deadlifts (2 Second Pause)	3		10	4		10	5		10	4		8	4		8	5		8
A3. Dumbbell 1 Arm Row	3		10	4		10	5		10	4		8	4		8	5		8
A4. Dumbbell Snatch	2		10	2		10	2		10	3		10	3		10	3		10
A5. Dumbbell Suit Case Carry (1 Arm)	2		30 Seconds Each Arm	2		35 Seconds Each Arm	2		40 Seconds Each Arm	3		45 Seconds Each Arm	3		55 Seconds Each Arm	3		60 Seconds Each Arm

Day 5	SETS	WT	REPS	SETS	WT	REPS	SETS	WT	REPS	SETS	WT	REPS	SETS	WT	REPS	SETS	WT	REPS
A1. Dumbbell Swing	3		10	4		10	5		10	3		15	4		15	5		15
A2. Dumbbell Push Press	3		8	4		8	5		8	3		12	4		12	5		12
A3. Dumbbell Goblet Squats (2 Second Pause)	3		5	4		5	5		5	3		12	4		12	5		10
A4. Dumbbell Hip Thrusts (2 Sec Pause)	3		12	4		12	5		12	4		15	4		15	5		20
A5. Dumbbell Farmers Walk (2 Arm)	3		30 Seconds Each Arm	3		35 Seconds Each Arm	3		40 Seconds Each Arm	3		45 Seconds Each Arm	3		55 Seconds Each Arm	3		60 Seconds Each Arm

Day 6 & 7 Rest/Active Recovery Day

Notes:

Barbell & Kettlebell Workout

STRENGTH TRAINING PLAN #4
Coach: Robert King

Barbell & Kettlebell - Strength, Muscle, Conditioning

Day 1	W1 SETS	W1 WT	W1 REPS	W2 SETS	W2 WT	W2 REPS	W3 SETS	W3 WT	W3 REPS	W4 SETS	W4 WT	W4 REPS	W5 SETS	W5 WT	W5 REPS	W6 SETS	W6 WT	W6 REPS
A1. Kettlebell Swing	3		10	4		10	5		10	3		15	4		8	5		8
B1. Barbell Squats	3		8	4		8	5		8	3		8	4		8	5		8
C1. Kettlebell Push Press	3		10	4		10	5		10	3		8	4		8	5		8
D1. Kettlebell Hip Thrusts	3		15	4		15	5		15	3		15	4		15	5		15
E1. Kettlebell Suit Case Carry (1 Arm)	3		30 Seconds Each Arm	3		35 Seconds Each Arm	3		40 Seconds Each Arm	3		45 Seconds Each Arm	3		55 Seconds Each Arm	3		60 Seconds Each Arm

Day 2	SETS	WT	REPS	SETS	WT	REPS	SETS	WT	REPS	SETS	WT	REPS	SETS	WT	REPS	SETS	WT	REPS
A1. Barbell Bench Press	3		8	4		8	5		8	3		10	5		10	5		10
B1. Kettlebell Snatch or KB Swing	3		8	4		8	5		8	3		10	5		10	5		10
C1. Barbell RDL (Romanian Deadlift)	3		8	4		8	5		8	3		10	5		10	5		10
D1. Kettlebell Hip Thrusts (2 Sec Pause)	3		12	4		12	4		12	4		15	5		15	5		15
E1. Kettlebell Farmers Walk (2 Arm)	3		30 Seconds Each Arm	3		35 Seconds Each Arm	3		40 Seconds Each Arm	3		45 Seconds Each Arm	3		55 Seconds Each Arm	3		60 Seconds Each Arm

Day 3 — Rest/ Active Recovery

Day 4	SETS	WT	REPS	SETS	WT	REPS	SETS	WT	REPS	SETS	WT	REPS	SETS	WT	REPS	SETS	WT	REPS
A1. Barbell Pause Squats	3		5	4		5	5		5	4		6	4		6	4		6
B1. Kettlebell Snatch or KB Swing	3		8	4		8	5		8	3		10	4		10	5		10
C1. Barbell Bent Over Row	3		10	4		10	5		10	4		8	4		8	5		8
D1. Barbell Hip Thrusts	3		10	4		10	5		10	3		10	4		10	5		10
E1. Kettlebell Suitcase Carry (1 Arm)	3		30 Seconds Each Arm	3		35 Seconds Each Arm	3		40 Seconds Each Arm	3		30 Seconds Each Arm	3		30 Seconds Each Arm	3		30 Seconds Each Arm

Day 5	SETS	WT	REPS	SETS	WT	REPS	SETS	WT	REPS	SETS	WT	REPS	SETS	WT	REPS	SETS	WT	REPS
A1. Kettlebell Swings	3		10	4		10	5		10	3		15	4		15	5		15
B1. Barbell Deadlifts	3		6	4		6	5		6	3		8	4		8	5		8
C1. Barbell Close Grip Bench Press (CG)	3		5	4		5	5		5	3		12	4		12	5		10
D1. Barbell Hip Thrusts 2 Second Pause	3		5	4		5	5		5	3		8	4		8	5		8
E1. Kettlebell Overhead Carry	3		30 Seconds Each Arm	3		35 Seconds Each Arm	3		40 Seconds Each Arm	3		30 Seconds Each Arm	3		30 Seconds Each Arm	3		30 Seconds Each Arm

Day 6 & 7 — Rest/Active Recovery Day

Notes:

Women Who Lift Weights
Coach: Robert King
info@womenwholiftweights_.com

Barbell & Dumbbell Workout

STRENGTH TRAINING PLAN #5

Barbell & Dumbbell - Strength & Muscle Hypertrophy

Coach: **Robert King**

	Week 1			Week 2			Week 3			Week 4			Week 5			Week 6		
Day 1	SETS	WT	REPS	SETS	WT	REPS	SETS	WT	REPS	SETS	WT	REPS	SETS	WT	REPS	SETS	WT	REPS
A1. Barbell Squats	3		8	4		8	5		8	3		8	4		8	5		8
A2. Dumbbell Push Press	3		8	4		8	5		8	3		8	4		8	5		8
B1. Dumbbell Bent Over Row	3		10	4		10	5		10	3		8	4		8	5		8
B2. Barbell Hip Thrusts	3		15	4		15	5		15	3		15	4		15	5		15
C1. Dumbbell Suit Case Carry (1 Arm)	3	30 Seconds Each Arm		3	35 Seconds Each Arm		3	40 Seconds Each Arm		3	45 Seconds Each Arm		3	50 Seconds Each Arm		3	60 Seconds Each Arm	
Day 2	SETS	WT	REPS	SETS	WT	REPS	SETS	WT	REPS	SETS	WT	REPS	SETS	WT	REPS	SETS	WT	REPS
A1. Barbell Bench Press	3		8	4		8	5		8	3		10	4		10	5		10
A2. Dumbbell RDL (Romanian Deadlift)	3		8	4		8	5		8	3		10	4		10	5		10
B1. Dumbbell Snatch	3		8	4		8	5		8	3		10	4		10	5		10
B2. Barbell Hip Thrusts (2 Sec Pause)	3		12	4		12	5		12	4		15	4		15	5		15
C1. Dumbbell Farmers Walk (2 Arm)	3	30 Seconds Each Arm		3	35 Seconds Each Arm		3	40 Seconds Each Arm		3	45 Seconds Each Arm		3	50 Seconds Each Arm		3	60 Seconds Each Arm	
Day 3	SETS	WT	REPS	SETS	WT	REPS	SETS	WT	REPS	SETS	WT	REPS	SETS	WT	REPS	SETS	WT	REPS
Rest/ Active Recovery																		
Day 4	SETS	WT	REPS	SETS	WT	REPS	SETS	WT	REPS	SETS	WT	REPS	SETS	WT	REPS	SETS	WT	REPS
A1. Barbell Pause Squats	3		5	4		5	5		5	4		6	4		6	5		6
A2. Dumbbell Military Press	3		8	4		8	5		8	3		10	4		10	5		10
B1. Barbell Bent Over Row	3		10	4		10	5		10	4		8	4		8	5		8
B2. Dumbbell Hip Thrusts	3		20	4		20	5		20	3		25	4		25	5		25
C1. Dumbbell Suitcase Carry (1 Arm)	3	30 Seconds Each Arm		3	35 Seconds Each Arm		3	40 Seconds Each Arm		3	45 Seconds Each Arm		3	50 Seconds Each Arm		3	60 Seconds Each Arm	
Day 5	SETS	WT	REPS	SETS	WT	REPS	SETS	WT	REPS	SETS	WT	REPS	SETS	WT	REPS	SETS	WT	REPS
A1. Barbell Deadlifts	3		6	4		6	5		6	3		8	4		8	5		8
B1. Dumbbell Walking Lunges	3		8	4		8	5		8	3		12	4		12	5		12
B2. Barbell Close Grip Bench Press (CG)	3		5	4		5	5		5	3		12	4		12	5		10
C1. Barbell Hip Thrusts 2 Second Pause	3		5	4		5	5		5	4		8	4		8	5		8
D1. Kettlebell Overhead Carry	3	30 Seconds Each Arm		3	35 Seconds Each Arm		3	40 Seconds Each Arm		3	45 Seconds Each Arm		3	50 Seconds Each Arm		3	60 Seconds Each Arm	
Day 6 & 7	SETS	WT	REPS	SETS	WT	REPS	SETS	WT	REPS	SETS	WT	REPS	SETS	WT	REPS	SETS	WT	REPS
Rest/Active Recovery Day																		

Notes:

Women Who Lift Weights

Coach: **Robert King**

info@womenwholiftweights.com

Kettlebell & Dumbbell Workout

STRENGTH TRAINING PLAN #6 Kettlebell & Dumbbell - Full Body Strength & Conditioning

Coach: Robert King

	Week 1			Week 2			Week 3			Week 4			Week 5			Week 6		
Day 1	SETS	WT	REPS	SETS	WT	REPS	SETS	WT	REPS	SETS	WT	REPS	SETS	WT	REPS	SETS	WT	REPS
A1. Kettlebell Squats	3		8	4		8	5		8	3		8	4		8	5		8
A2. Dumbbell Push Press	3		8	4		8	5		8	3		8	4		8	5		8
B1. Dumbbell Bent Over Row	3		10	4		10	5		10	3		8	4		8	5		8
B2. Kettlebell Hip Thrusts	3		15	4		15	5		15	3		15	4		15	5		15
C1. Dumbbell Suit Case Carry (1 Arm)	3		30 Seconds Each Arm	3		35 Seconds Each Arm	3		40 Seconds Each Arm	3		45 Seconds Each Arm	3		50 Seconds Each Arm	3		60 Seconds Each Arm
Day 2	SETS	WT	REPS	SETS	WT	REPS	SETS	WT	REPS	SETS	WT	REPS	SETS	WT	REPS	SETS	WT	REPS
A1. KB Swings	3		8	4		8	5		8	3		10	4		10	5		10
A2. DB Push Press	3		8	4		8	5		8	3		10	4		10	5		10
B1. Dumbbell Snatch	3		8	4		8	5		8	3		10	4		10	5		10
B2. Kettlebell Deadlift	3		8	4		8	5		8	4		10	4		10	5		10
C1. Dumbbell Farmers Walk (2 Arm)	3		30 Seconds Each Arm	3		35 Seconds Each Arm	3		40 Seconds Each Arm	3		45 Seconds Each Arm	3		50 Seconds Each Arm	3		60 Seconds Each Arm
Day 3	SETS	WT	REPS	SETS	WT	REPS	SETS	WT	REPS	SETS	WT	REPS	SETS	WT	REPS	SETS	WT	REPS
Rest/ Active Recovery																		
Day 4	SETS	WT	REPS	SETS	WT	REPS	SETS	WT	REPS	SETS	WT	REPS	SETS	WT	REPS	SETS	WT	REPS
A1. Kettlebell Goblet Pause Squats	3		8	4		8	5		8	4		10	4		10	5		10
A2. Dumbbell Military Press	3		8	4		8	5		8	3		10	4		10	5		10
B1. Dumbbell Bent Over Row	3		10	4		10	5		10	4		8	4		8	5		8
B2. Kettlebell Swings	3		10	4		10	5		10	3		15	4		15	5		15
C1. Kettlebell Suit Case Carry (1 Arm)	3		30 Seconds Each Arm	3		35 Seconds Each Arm	3		40 Seconds Each Arm	3		45 Seconds Each Arm	3		50 Seconds Each Arm	3		60 Seconds Each Arm
Day 5	SETS	WT	REPS	SETS	WT	REPS	SETS	WT	REPS	SETS	WT	REPS	SETS	WT	REPS	SETS	WT	REPS
A1. Kettlebell Deadlifts	3		10	4		10	5		10	3		12	4		12	5		12
B1. Dumbbell Walking Lunges	3		8	4		8	5		8	3		12	4		12	5		12
B2. Kettlebell or DB Military Press	3		5	4		5	5		5	3		12	4		12	5		10
C1. KB or DB Hip Thrusts 2 Second Pause	3		10	4		10	5		10	3		15	4		15	5		15
C2. Kettlebell Farmers Walk (2 Arm)	3		30 Seconds Each Arm	3		35 Seconds Each Arm	3		40 Seconds Each Arm	3		45 Seconds Each Arm	3		50 Seconds Each Arm	3		60 Seconds Each Arm
Day 6 & Day 7	SETS	WT	REPS	SETS	WT	REPS	SETS	WT	REPS	SETS	WT	REPS	SETS	WT	REPS	SETS	WT	REPS
Rest/Active Recovery Day																		

Women Who Lift Weights

Coach: Robert King

info@womenwholiftweights.com

Notes:

Barbell, Kettlebell & Dumbbell Workout

STRENGTH TRAINING PLAN #7   Barbell + Kettlebell + Dumbbell – Strength, Muscle, Conditioning

Coach: Robert King

Day 1

Exercise	W1 Sets	W1 Reps	W2 Sets	W2 Reps	W3 Sets	W3 Reps	W4 Sets	W4 Reps	W5 Sets	W5 Reps	W6 Sets	W6 Reps
A1. Kettlebell Swing	3	10	4	10	5	10	3	15	5	8	5	8
A2. Barbell Squats	3	8	4	8	5	8	3	8	5	8	5	8
B1. Dumbbell Push Press	3	10	4	10	5	10	3	8	5	8	5	8
B2. Barbell or DB Rows	3	10	4	10	5	10	3	12	5	12	5	12
C1. Barbell Hip Thrusts	3	10	4	10	5	10	3	10	5	10	5	10
C2. Kettlebell Suit Case Carry (1 Arm)	3	30 Seconds Each Arm	3	35 Seconds Each Arm	3	40 Seconds Each Arm	3	45 Seconds Each Arm	3	55 Seconds Each Arm	3	60 Seconds Each Arm

Day 2

Exercise	W1 Sets	W1 Reps	W2 Sets	W2 Reps	W3 Sets	W3 Reps	W4 Sets	W4 Reps	W5 Sets	W5 Reps	W6 Sets	W6 Reps
A1. Barbell or DB OH Press	3	8	4	8	5	8	3	10	5	10	5	10
B1. Barbell or DB Romanian Deadlifts	3	8	4	8	5	8	3	10	5	10	5	10
C1 Barbell RDL (Romanian Deadlift)	3	8	4	8	5	8	3	10	5	10	5	10
D1. Kettlebell Hip Thrusts (2 Sec Pause)	3	12	4	12	5	12	4	15	4	15	5	15
E1. Kettlebell Farmers Walk (2 Arm)	3	30 Seconds Each Arm	3	35 Seconds Each Arm	3	40 Seconds Each Arm	3	45 Seconds Each Arm	3	55 Seconds Each Arm	3	60 Seconds Each Arm

Day 3

Rest/ Active Recovery

Day 4

Exercise	W1 Sets	W1 Reps	W2 Sets	W2 Reps	W3 Sets	W3 Reps	W4 Sets	W4 Reps	W5 Sets	W5 Reps	W6 Sets	W6 Reps
A1. Barbell or DB Bench Press/Floor Press	3	5	4	5	5	5	4	6	4	6	5	6
B1. Kettlebell Snatch or KB Swing	3	8	4	8	5	8	3	10	4	10	5	10
C1. Barbell Bent Over Row	3	10	4	10	5	10	4	8	4	8	5	8
D1. Barbell Hip Thrusts	3	10	4	10	5	10	3	10	3	10	5	10
E1. Dumbbell Suitcase Carry (1 Arm)	3	30 Seconds Each Arm	3	35 Seconds Each Arm	3	40 Seconds Each Arm	3	30 Seconds Each Arm	3	30 Seconds Each Arm	3	30 Seconds Each Arm

Day 5

Exercise	W1 Sets	W1 Reps	W2 Sets	W2 Reps	W3 Sets	W3 Reps	W4 Sets	W4 Reps	W5 Sets	W5 Reps	W6 Sets	W6 Reps
A1. Kettlebell Swings	3	10	4	10	5	10	3	15	4	15	5	15
B1. Barbell Deadlifts	3	6	4	6	5	6	3	8	4	8	5	8
C1 Barbell Close Grip Bench Press (CG)	3	5	4	5	5	5	3	8	4	8	5	8
D1. Barbell Hip Thrusts 2 Second Pause	3	8	4	8	5	8	4	12	4	12	5	12
E1. Dumbbell Farmers Carry 2 arm	3	30 Seconds Each Arm	3	35 Seconds Each Arm	3	40 Seconds Each Arm	3	30 Seconds Each Arm	3	30 Seconds Each Arm	3	30 Seconds Each Arm

Day 6 & Day 7

Rest/Active Recovery Day

Notes:

Women Who Lift Weights

info@womenwholiftweights.com

Coach: Robert King

CHAPTER 13

MYTHS OF WOMEN'S STRENGTH TRAINING

It's vital that you learn some of the key mistakes that most women do make when starting out with a strength-training program. While it's great that you are excited about this exercise and getting started on it, if you are making these major errors, you are most definitely going to influence the results that you see.

Women and men share some common mistakes in strength training, However men have some common flaws that are different from women.

Often men don't spend enough time building a strong technical foundation, they rely more on "muscling the weights" with strength. Another issue is that a lot of men lack patience and often add too much weight too fast which leads to burn out, injury and more.

If you want to experience maximum success, you need to be using the right overall workout setup — one that will strengthen the body and help you burn fat, not just waste your time in the gym.

Let's take a look at the most important things to note.

Not Lifting Sufficient Weight

The very first big problem that often occurs is that you are not using sufficient weigh to stimulate your muscles maximally. Again, this tends to go back to the fact that you are scared that heavy weights will make you too 'muscular.'

This really isn't the case.

Realize that it's only heavy weight that will overload the body and that overload is what is really needed in order to change your body.

If you aren't applying a heavy weight during the workout, you're really doing little more than just burning off some calories.

It's when you apply the heavy weight that you shock the muscles. This will create tiny muscle tears that they have to recover from and then grow back stronger than you were before.

If you're supplying a resistance with a lighter weight that the muscles can easily already tolerate, then what reason do they have to change?

They can already sufficiently handle that weight so there is no reason to change at all. They are fine just the way they are.

But you are not fine with your body just the way it is; thus, you will be disappointed in the results that you get.

Performing High Rep Training

The second major mistake that many women make whenn going about a strength-training workout program is performing far too much higher rep training.

You know the type – the 'toning' workout sets.

You take the rep range up to around 15 to 25, thinking this will help you burn calories and tone those muscles.

Here again, note that if you're able to do 15 to 25 reps at a given weight on an exercise, all that means is that this weight is not challenging you nearly enough.

As a general guideline, you should never be able to go beyond about 12 reps on any exercise that you do. If you can, you're not going to get benefits from that working set.

Lower rep training is what will boost the metabolism more, stimulate greater overall strength gains, and create the body-changing benefits that you're looking for.

Not Resting Enough

Another vital mistake that cannot be made if you're going to see maximum results from your training is not getting sufficient rest.

Many, many women suffer from this because they adopt the mindset that 'more is better.' You're on a mission to lose those last stubborn ten pounds and that means getting into the gym each and every day for at least an hour.

You are there to burn calories — even if it kills you.

What you must realize here, especially when it comes to strength training, is that your body does require so much rest.

If you don't rest and allow the recovery process to take place, you're virtually just going to keep tearing down the muscle cells further and further, growing weaker and weaker in the process.

Rest is when you actually grow back stronger than you were before, so if you're skipping over rest, you're basically just moving backwards rather than forwards.

Also note that especially with women, some very strange things tend to happen when not enough rest is given and you start moving into a realm of overtraining.

When too much exercise is combined with too few calories coming in, the body moves deep into that state of being overtrained. The metabolism slows down and your body starts retaining a whole lot of excess water.

What this is going to do is give you a very bloated, puffy-looking appearance — one that you definitely did not have in mind when setting your goals.

Many women often suffer from this training-induced water retention along with inflammation and then it appears as though you aren't losing any weight at all.

In fact, you may even be *gaining* weight.

When you finally take some time off and allow your body a full recovery from those hard workout sessions, like magic you begin losing weight again and start looking leaner than you have in years.

When it comes to creating an attractive-looking body, too much training is never a good thing. You may think the more exercise you do the better you'll get, but the body can only handle so much before it's virtually like 'all systems shut down.'

You'll feel tired, you'll feel irritable, and you'll have a metabolic rate that's just crawling along at a snail's pace.

Not Fuelling Your Body

Finally, the last big mistake that many females make as they go about their training is not fuelling your body.

This issue comes about due to years and years of trying to lose weight and being put on restrictive diet after restrictive diet.

Most women, by nature, are natural food restrictors. You aren't eating enough calories to even maintain your weight with no activity, not to mention all the additional workout sessions added in.

Again, this creates problems because not only is your body not getting the fuel reserves it needs to recover from those intense training workout sessions, it's not getting enough to maximize the metabolic rate either.

So, over time the metabolism starts to get more and more sluggish, making it harder and harder for you to see the weight loss results you desire.

As we mentioned earlier, due to the fact that you are weight training, you will be setting your body up for being able to handle a few more calories each day because you'll have that muscle glycogen storage that the calories can go into. You'll also have a slightly higher resting metabolic rate as well.

So there really is no reason to go to the extremes and cut your calories way back when you have all these benefits working in your favour.

There you have the main mistakes that many women make with their weight training program. Obviously, the biggest mistake is not even getting started on a problem in the first place, but when that program is in place, then these are the mistakes that are most commonly seen and the ones that you must be on the lookout for if you are going to see optimal success.

So now that you know what you shouldn't be doing, let's move forward and begin going over what you should be doing for the best body-changing results.

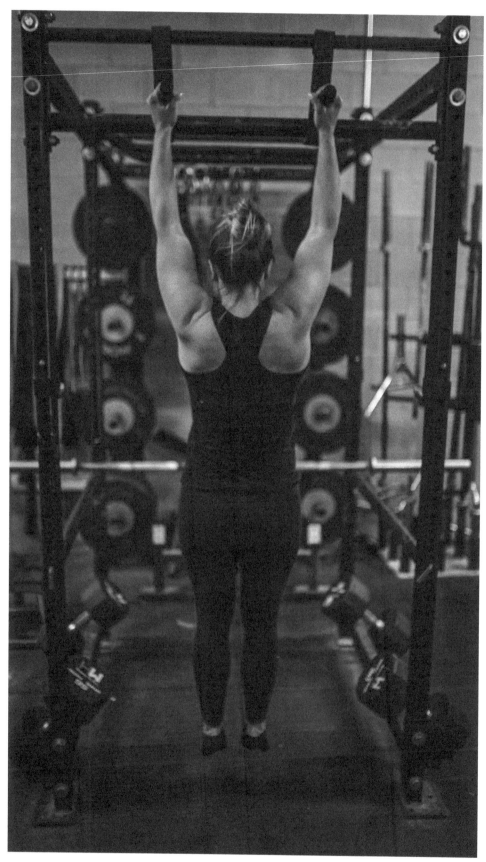

Nancy Pull Up

CHAPTER 14

EIGHT TRAINING DIFFERENCES BETWEEN WOMEN AND MEN

When it comes to lifting weights and getting stronger, there are general rules that apply to both men and women.

However, there are subtle differences when it comes to how women should train for maximal results compared to men.

Here are a few training differences that are worth noting for women compared to men.

1. Less Rest Time Between Sets

Women require less rest time between sets than men. Give a woman three-plus minutes between sets and oftentimes she will be bored beyond belief.

I have to time my female strength athletes to make sure they take enough adequate rest time as women usually feel like they need to do something all the time. Resting and recovering while lifting weights is very important.

What you can do during "rest" time, as rest is needed, is a non-demanding exercise.

For example, let's say you are doing barbell back squats and you need five minutes of rest between sets. At about the half way point of the rest, you can add in a dumbbell push press or a box jump. Do something that won't be demanding on the legs or the nervous system.

I would not recommend any cardio or high intensity exercises during this rest. The goal is to get better, get stronger, not get tired.

This keeps workouts exciting and also offers better time utilization.

2. More Sets

Women can handle a much larger workload of sets than men. I can hit my female clients with 10 sets in a 30-minute workout and they are fine. Try getting guys to do this and they will struggle big time.

However, while women seem to be able to handle lower body volume very well, this is not as much the case when it comes to upper body volume.

3. More Frequent Training

Women tend to recover faster and can train more days per week than men. Some of the top women I coached for all levels of athletics trained five-plus days a week. Most times I am encouraging my female athletes to rest more, which they have trouble doing.

4. The Importance of Technique While Lifting

I have met some women who are naturally just strong — you know, brutish-type strength.

But most of the women who are strong in the gym are strong technically and mentally.

To be strong in the gym, it's not about raw strength; it's about technique, practice, and hard work. For a woman to lift heavy weights, technique is always very important.

5. Importance Of "The Kaizen Principle" for Women Lifting

According to the Kaizen principle, slow and steady gains over long periods of time add up. A female can hit a 250-pound deadlift and go to 255 pounds and it can be nailed to the floor. Know your numbers and take small improvements over time.

6. The Need For Grip Strength

Every woman I have trained became stronger overall once their grip improved. I know this could also be applied to men, but overall grip strength is something that females tend to lack when starting lifting. Once grip improves, things in the gym improve fast.

One of the simplest things you can do to improve grip is do weighted carries and thick grip training. If you are not doing these two simple things, then you are not as strong as you can be.

Grab a set of these thick grips and use these in your accessory work and arm day.

Weak grip is usually a limiting factor in women's strength that can be fixed with a bit of work and direct grip training.

7. Women are Generally More "Coachable"

Women are much easier to coach than men.

Women generally are more coachable and listen better to coaching (not all, keep in mind).

Men are more stubborn when it comes to lifting weights. Most men seem to like pump-type workouts and machines. In contrast, many women love strength once they are taught how to lift properly.

Women love learning about strength and technique.

8. Mindset Training for Women

I coach my female clients very differently than I coach my male clients. For lifting, guys can use aggression and anger a lot more than women can.

With my female clients I have to "trick them" a lot when it comes to lifting. I do not tell them what is on the bar. Once a female lifter trusts that you believe she can lift the weight, there is a MUCH higher chance she will make the lift.

Guys often think they can lift more than they can; women far too often underestimate what they are capable of doing.

CHAPTER 15

CONNECT WITH COACH ROB & WWLW

I hope that you found that this book helped you in many ways.

Thank you for allowing me to share my passion of strength training and lifting weights with you.

If you found this book helpful or even if you just want to say hi and connect, I would love to hear from you.

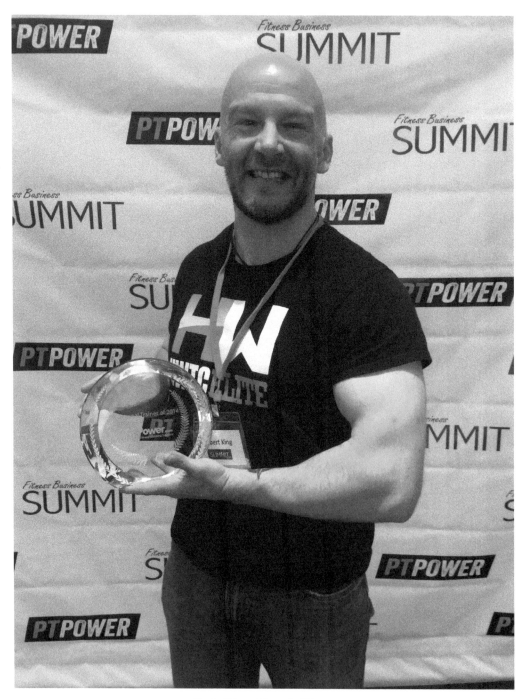

Rob King Coach Shot

Coach Rob King Contact Info:

✉ at Robkingfitness@gmail.com

📷 www.Instagram.com/CoachRobertKing (@CoachRobertKing)

f www.Facebook.com/RobKingFitness

🏀 www.RobKingFitness.com

Women Who Lift Weights Info:

✉ at Info@womenwholiftweights.com

📷 www.Instagram.com/WomenWhoLiftWeights (@WomenWhoLiftWeights)

f www.Facebook.com/groups/WomenWhoLiftWeights

🏀 www.WomenWhoLiftWeights.com

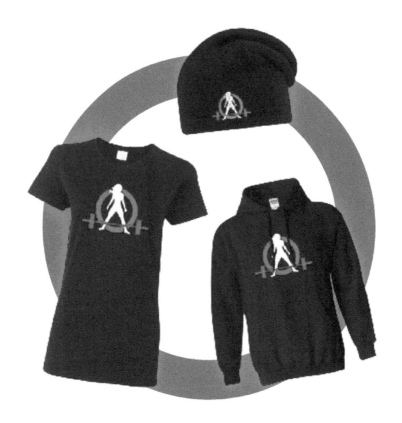

Check Out Our WWLW Shop

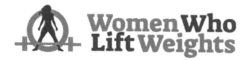
Shop Now

 @womenwholiftweights

 @womenwholiftweights

 info@womenwholiftweights.com

 www.womenwholiftweights.com

Lightning Source UK Ltd.
Milton Keynes UK
UKHW050255220222
399010UK00005B/284

9 780228 849759